Teaching Reiki

A Comprehensive Guide to Running Great Courses

by Taggart King

*To Dear Helen,
With Reiki hugs!
TAGGART
X*

www.reiki-evolution.co.uk

taggart@reiki-evolution.co.uk

ISBN 978-1-9998852-1-2

3

Introduction

This is the book that I wish had been available when I first started running Reiki courses… and I wish it had been available when I had been running courses for some time, actually!

What I have tried to do is to bring together in one place a lot of useful and practical information about setting up and running Reiki courses.

I start by including a range of articles about different aspects of teaching Reiki: reminding you about how much you already know and explaining how to plan and structure your courses, then moving on to talk about what to say and how to say it when you explain things to and guide your students, including how to make sure your courses deal with students' individual learning styles and personality types.

Then I move on to explain how to create your own course materials (manuals and audio CDs) and how to support your students long-term, whether through hosting Reiki 'shares', running Reiki 'practice' days or in other ways.

Having put those basic building blocks in place, we move on to the actual courses themselves, and because one thing is common to all Reiki courses – the Reiki initiations – I talk for a little while about what we actually do when we 'attune' someone to Reiki, what attunements you should use, how many you need to carry out, and how Reiju empowerments fit in to the picture.

Now, obviously, my experience involves putting together "Reiki Evolution" style courses, which are a lot more focused on original Japanese Reiki – what Mikao Usui was teaching in the early years of the 20th century – than the more standard "Western style" Reiki courses, which derive from the teachings of Dr Hayashi, as passed on to the West by Mrs Takata, and endlessly mutated thereafter.

So I detail what we know about the Reiki that Usui Sensei was teaching, compare that with the contents of most Western-style Reiki courses, and show how I have put together my courses, to include as much as is practical of the original system, while still following a weekend-course form of teaching (rather than a 'dojo' format) and retaining, with a Japanese twist, the main Western Reiki approaches.

I suggest a course schedule for the three Reiki levels – First Degree, Second Degree and Master level (or a Master/Teacher course, as it is referred to in some quarters) and go into a lot of detail about what to say and what practical exercises to go through with your students, if you were going to teach "Reiki Evolution style".

Finally, I talk about my experience of teaching Reiki First and Second Degree in a ten-week 'evening class' format, showing how I structured the courses, what I taught and when, and I include the text of ten A4 hand-outs that I gave to students.

I hope that, no matter what your Reiki lineage or style of Reiki, there will be little nuggets of good advice and useful ideas in this book which you can use straight away to benefit your Reiki students, whether that means giving you the confidence to realise that you **can** run your own courses, helping you to enhance the effectiveness of your teaching and improve the quality of your course materials, or helping you to provide better or more creative long-term support to the people that you have trained.

Teaching Reiki is – or certainly should be – a long journey of continuous self-reflection and improvement, where you look at what you are doing, take note of positive and negative feedback from your students, and make your courses better, again and again and again.

Introducing someone to Reiki can have such a profound and life-changing effect on a person, and we are in such a lucky position to play a part in helping that process get underway. We owe it to our students to provide them with the very best we are capable of and I hope that this book goes some way to helping you with your own journey of 'kaizen', of never-ending improvement.

With my very best wishes, and a big Reiki hug.

Taggart King

www.reiki-evolution.co.uk

GENERAL ADVICE ABOUT REIKI COURSES AND TEACHING

Advice for new Reiki teachers

It's nerve-wracking preparing for your first Reiki course, isn't it? You're taking a step into the unknown and you are going to be guiding a group of people who are trusting you to do a good job. You probably feel that you don't know enough and that you're not ready yet. I know how that feels.

I this article I thought I would just pass on a few pieces of advice that might be of help to you, to ease some of your anxiety. Here goes...

It's OK to teach differently from how you were taught

I'm sure that the First Degree course you went on was great and gave you everything you needed. But the course may be a bit hazy now, given that you have gone on to take Second Degree and your Master Teacher course.

Maybe you have a sense that you would like to do things a bit differently from the way that your teacher taught you: you are a different person, you have a different personality, you approach things in different ways.

And that's ok: you should not feel that you have to exactly replicate the way that they taught or the content

11

of their course. You can be yourself and find your own distinctive way, so long as you pass on the essentials, which you can read about in this article: Back to basics: all about Reiki First Degree. So if you think you can explain things better, provide better course materials, or think the course would flow more logically if you did things differently, go right ahead.

Teach Reiki, not stuff that has nothing to do with Reiki

This is a bit of a bug-bear of mine, but I shall say it anyway: make sure that when you teach Reiki, you just teach Reiki, rather than a whole load of New-Age add-ons that have very little or nothing to do with Usui Reiki but have crept into Reiki over the years, and here I am thinking about smudging, crystal healing, chakra balancing, tarot cards, spirit guides and clairvoyance. When you run a Reiki course, I recommend that you teach Reiki, just Reiki.

Make sure that you have practised your attunements well

No matter what lineage you have, you are going to carry out some initiations with your students, whether that be Reiju empowerments or some other variety of attunement ritual. You need to be comfortable in giving these initiations because you don't want to have to keep flicking through your notes half way through the attunements. That would be so unprofessional.

So practise, practise and practise some more!

Attune a teddy bear, attune an empty chair, sit in your lounge on a sofa with your eyes closed and imagine in your mind's eye you giving an attunement, see yourself going through the movements, explain out loud what you are doing (as if you were explaining to someone else how to do it), gesticulate so you get used to the hand movements, walk up and down like a mad person, talking yourself through the stages you have learned, draw little stick-figure diagrams to summarise the stages, rap a little rhyme to remind your mind! Be creative!

Once you have the attunements sorted you will feel a lot more confident.

You don't need to have all the answers

You are probably worrying about what people might ask you on your course and whether you will know the answer to all their questions. You probably think that you don't know enough.

To be honest, so long as you know more than they do then you will be fine, and you know far more than you think. Your students don't really know anything about Reiki and you have been using it for some time now, so you have a wealth of experience to draw upon.

But there's more to say about questions because you do not have to have the answer to every question; I know I don't.

Some questions do not have an answer, or nobody knows, or nobody knows and it doesn't matter anyway.

Don't waffle or try to make up an answer: people can tell if you're bullshitting, and if you're honest with your students then they will take more notice of you when you do have something to say.

Remember that Reiki is a practical art

Remember that Reiki is a practical art and that when you teach Reiki you are passing on what you have learned and noticed during your personal experience of working with the energy. You are not passing on high-blown academic theories that you have to revise and might get wrong: you have personal experience of doing all the things that you will be guiding your students through, so you are on very solid ground.

You have given yourself a lot of self-treatments and if you learned Japanese-style Reiki then you will also have experience of using Hatsurei ho most days, and working with the Reiki precepts. You have given Reiki treatments to other people and you have become comfortable with this, learning from your experiences and finding your own comfortable way with the process, making it your own.

You know far, far more about all this stuff than they do, you know far more than you realise, and you have personal experience of doing all the things that you will be guiding your students through… so you can chill, be yourself, and enjoy the day.

And I am sure that you will have a wonderful time on your course.

Reiki teaching: what are your goals?

When you are starting to teach Reiki courses and are planning what you are going to cover, demonstrate and say, it is very important that you start with a clear idea of what you're aiming for: your goals.

Goals can encompass what information you want your students to have taken on board and understood, what practical exercises you want them to have been through, and feel comfortable with, and what 'Reiki worldview' you want to instil. I will talk more about this last item further down the page.

Knowledge goals

Most teachers will want their students to have a fairly good idea about:

- What Reiki is
- Where it comes from
- What Reiki can do for them if they work with the energy and the precepts regularly
- What Reiki can do for other people when they receive Reiki treatments

This information can be made available on a web site, so potential students can find out about these areas even before they book on a course. So, for example, the

"About Reiki Healing" page of the Reiki Evolution web site starts with this text:

Reiki is a simple Japanese energy system anyone can learn

- Experience peace of mind and inner calm
- Relieve stress and anxiety
- Bring a sense of balance and wholeness
- Help family and friends
- Explore your spiritual side
- Let go of emotional baggage

Further down the page I include links that people can follow to find out more about a whole range of issues to do with Reiki.

If you have your own web site and would like to be able to refer to these articles, please include a link from your web site to any of these pages. Don't copy and paste the text into your own site, though, because Google won't like that and will penalise your site.

Then the information can be repeated, rewritten or summarised in your course materials (your manual, maybe on an audio CD).

You will see in my article "Reiki teaching: your course materials" that I recommend that you send your course materials out to your students in advance so they can take their time and mull over this information, and re-visit it several times before arriving on your course, and this means that they day of your course can involve you just re-capping the main points, rather than trying to tell everyone everything, for the first time, on a course where your students are half-zonked-out on the energy and in the worst position to be able to assimilate new information!

How to work out what to tell them

There is a lot of information out there to do with Reiki and it can be difficult sometimes to see the wood for the trees. What do you tell them? What should you start with?

To get some focus, ask yourself this question for each category of information (what Reiki is, where Reiki comes from, What Reiki can do for you etc):

1. If I could only tell my students five things, what would they be?
2. If I had to blurt out the basic info in a 30 second conversation with someone while travelling in a lift, what would I blurt out?

These questions give you an idea of the priorities, the main themes, and then you can expand on these themes and provide additional supporting info and examples. I talk more about this in my article "Reiki teaching: explain, guide and review".

Practical goals

Here is where you decide what practical exercises you want your students to go through on your course, what they need to feel comfortable with, and what they need to understand about what they are doing.

For a First Degree course you might want to focus on:

- Experiencing energy between your hands and around someone else's hands
- Feeling energy around someone else's head and shoulders
- Carrying out Hatsurei ho
- Performing a self-treatment
- Practising scanning
- Giving a full treatment
- Receiving a full treatment

For a Second Degree course you might focus on:

- Experiencing the energy of earth ki
- Experiencing the energy of heavenly ki
- Using these two energies to treat someone
- Sending distant healing so you can start to experience oneness
- Practising working intuitively
- Exploring use power of intent through visualisation

For each of these, decide what you want them to do, precisely, and how you are going to explain and talk people through these exercises? Work out what you need to the student to understand about what they did. What do these exercises mean for them, why are they important, how will they use them in practice and what might they notice when they carry out these exercises in the coming weeks and months?

More 'global' goals

In a wider sense, my goal is to create independent Reiki practitioners who are comfortable working with the energy, flexible and intuitive in their approach, not attached to dogma, not judgmental of other people's different ways of practising Reiki, and not dependent on me as a teacher to dispense all the answers.

I hope that they should be able to embrace uncertainty, following a Reiki path as a journey of self-development, not believing that what they were taught is the 'one true way' or the 'absolute truth'.

In my blog "My Manifesto for Reiki Tolerance" I spoke about how Reiki is a very flexible and accommodating system and acts as a 'carrier' that accommodates very many different ways of working, some simple, some more complex. I spoke about how some ways of working naturally attract some people, while for others a different way of working feels more 'right' for them.

I hope that my students will not treat the Reiki Evolution approach as 'the one true way' and look down on or disparage other practitioners' methods, even though it is not uncommon for some Reiki people to behave in this way.

I want to promote tolerance and respect and compassion for others and I believe that they way that I and my team of teachers speak about Reiki promotes this.

Structuring your Reiki course

At Reiki Evolution we have a steady stream of students coming to us to re-take their Reiki courses because they weren't very happy with their original Reiki training, and we hear quite a few horror stories about wholly inadequate Reiki training courses.

The main criticisms fall into three categories:

- Aimless drifting through the day of the course, talking about things unrelated to Reiki
- Emerging from the course without a clear idea of what Reiki is or how to use it
- Hardly any hands-on practice at actually doing Reiki, but a lot of talking

So if a student ends up spending their time on a course sipping herb tea while chatting randomly about what everyone thinks of Reflexology or what the last Natural Healing Exhibition everyone went to was like, as if there was no time pressure at all, drifting through the day not really finding out very much about Reiki and not having much of an opportunity to try doing Reiki, that course is not good enough.

You would be surprised to find out how many courses are actually like that, and you need to make sure that you do not end up hosting such an unstructured and poor quality course yourself!

You need a definite structure

Effective Reiki courses need to have a definite structure, where the teacher knows in advance what they are going to say, what they are going to demonstrate, what exercises and practices they are going to talk their students through, and what they aim for their students to know and be able to do by the end of the course.

You set a schedule and stick to it because if you spend an hour too much on one particular task or practice then you end up rushing, and skimping, on another area. You need to keep an eye on the time, and stick to your schedule as far as is practical.

Work out what you are going to cover in the morning, and what you are going to cover in the afternoon. Give your students a definite mid-morning break, at a definite time, so you break the morning, and the afternoon for that matter, into two separate sessions, and give your students a definite lunch break; I think lunch should be at least 45 minutes.

Students need a chance to get out of the room, get some fresh air and maybe go for a bit of a walk to clear their heads

In your pre-planned sessions you're there to talk about, demonstrate and supervise people practising Reiki.

In your scheduled breaks you can chat about whatever you like, and remember that you need to have a decent break for lunch, too, to clear your head and get some fresh air and a change of scenery.

Reiki Evolution First Degree courses

As an example, here's a list of the 'main headings' from our Reiki First Degree courses:

- Introduction
- Reiju empowerment #1
- Practice: Experiencing energy
- Reiju empowerment #2
- Practice: Daily energy exercises
- Reiju empowerment #3
- Practice: Self-treatments

LUNCH

- Talk/Demo: Treating other people
- Practice: feeling the energy field
- Practice: scanning
- Practice: give and receive a full treatment

You can see that in our morning session, the students receive their three Reiki initiations, they are introduced to the idea of energy and given the chance to feel energy for the first time, they learn how to carry out some daily energy exercises (Hatsurei ho) and they are guided through a form of self-treatment (in this case, the self-treatment meditation that Usui Sensei taught).

22

The afternoon session moves on from working on yourself to working on other people, with the teacher giving a talk and brief demonstration of a Reiki treatment, showing hand positions, giving hints and tips, and then students practise working with energy again, this time feeling another student's energy field and trying out 'scanning' for the first time. This leads on to the giving and receiving of a full treatment.

Reiki is a practical skill

You will have noticed that there is a lot of hands-on practice in this schedule. There is a good reason for this: Reiki is a practical skill, and you learn a skill by doing it, not just hearing about it. You can't learn to swim by attending lectures about swimming: you have to get in the water and do it, with advice and guidance from your instructor.

It's not enough to tell them what to do: they need to have had practical experience of actually doing the things they will do when using Reiki for themselves and others.

Our aim is for our students to come out of our First Degree course with a clear idea of what Reiki is, where it comes from, and how they can use it simply to work on themselves and treat other people

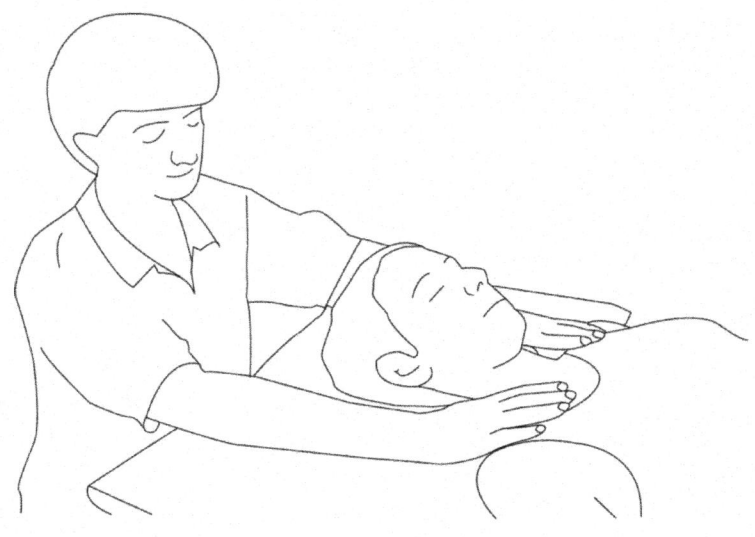

They will have experienced energy in different ways,
practised a self-treatment, used Hatsurei ho and they
will have given and received a full Reiki treatment.

These are the essential components of a Reiki First
Degree course. You can read more about what Reiki 1
should be about by reading my blog entitled "Back to
basics: all about Reiki First Degree", which you can find
reproduced later in this book, when I talk in detail about
teaching Reiki First Degree.

Reiki teaching: explain, guide and review

When you teach someone Reiki, you are teaching a practical skill, an art. Reiki is about things that you do: you meditate, you move energy with visualisation or intention, you move through hand positions as you treat other people, and students need to become comfortable with these practical skills by doing them: initially on their Reiki course and then through repeated practice once they get back home, in the days and weeks after their course.

It occurred to me that when I teach Reiki I go through a particular sequence, with the students sitting in front of me, whenever I teach a particular practice, and you can summarise what I do with these headings:

1. Explain
2. Guide
3. Review

Explain

You need to explain clearly to your students what it is that they will be doing: what the stages are, how they will do it.

Maybe you need to demonstrate a few points, or a few movements, and have your students copy you a few times so that they are comfortable with the process, before they do it 'for real'.

Reassure them that they don't need to remember anything at this stage because you will talk them through the process.

Talk about why you do this exercise, what it is said to achieve and what they might notice, reassuring them that everyone is different and that you are not expecting people to experience a particular thing: that there is no 'right' thing that they have to notice.

Guide

Most of the things that we do when we practise Reiki, we do with our eyes closed: meditating, self-treating, performing Hatsurei ho, treating other people, so we need to be guided through these practices for the first time, by a teacher who is paying close attention to us, and who explains what we need to do clearly and carefully, moving everyone through the stages at the same time.

Review

When you have completed an exercise, ask the students what they noticed, what they enjoyed, what they found challenging, how it went for them.

You don't necessarily have to go round eliciting feedback in order, say from right to left, because that might be intimidating for the first person you keep on coming to.

Just allow the person who feels most comfortable giving their feedback to do so first, but also make sure that you ask everyone what they experienced, so everyone has the chance to share.

It is useful for students to understand that there are differences in their experiences when carrying out a particular exercise and that is ok: everyone is different and experiences things in different ways.

And if everyone noticed a particular thing happening, then that's great too!

Feedback is useful because it often raises issues, or questions, that you can use as 'talking points' where you can provide further advice, or practical tips, or talk about perhaps different ways that the exercises can be used (for example, taking Kenyoku out of Hatsurei ho and using it before treating someone).

And if no-one asks the question that would lead you to give that helpful hint or tip, give them the tips anyway.

Explain, Guide, Review, Repeat

You can cycle through these three stages for each chunk of your course: each practical exercise.

So before you give the first attunement or empowerment, explain what you are doing and why, and what they are going to have to do to participate (for example, "bring your hands into the prayer position when I rest my hand gently on your shoulder"), go through the initiation, let them know when you have completed the process for everyone, and get feedback about what people noticed.

When you teach Hatsurei ho, talk about why you do this exercise, the stages they need to go through, the movements that they will need to make (let them practise a few times), guide them through the exercise in real time and then ask for feedback so you can provide useful hints and tips, reassurance, and talk about how the exercise, or parts of the exercise, can be used in different situations.

And so on for self-treatments and treating other people.

On a Second Degree course, for example, you can use the same sequence to introduce meditations on the energies of earth ki and heavenly ki, to deal with distant healing and working intuitively.

Reiki teaching: tell them, tell them and tell them

In my article "Reiki teaching: explain, guide, review" I ran through a simple sequence that you can follow when teaching practical exercises to your students.

In this article I would like to talk about the information that you pass on, how to help the information to stick in your students' minds, and how to ensure that new information relates to what has come before, and is put in proper context.

And in doing this, I will be relying on some very basic advice that is given to people who do public speaking. In fact, this is the most basic public speaking advice!

How to speak in public

When you give a talk to a group of people, you need to:

1. Tell them what you are going to tell them
2. Tell them
3. Tell them what you told them

So you have an introduction where you run over the main themes or areas that you are going to be covering. This starts to give your listeners a 'map of the territory',

29

it provides them with a set of main headings or categories, so when you move on to the next stage ('tell them') you can expand on those themes and headings.

The listener already has some 'hooks' in their memory to add the new information to, so it makes sense, has somewhere to fit, and will be more memorable.

Finally, you tell them what you told them, which means that, after having explored the issues in detail, you conclude by bringing them back to the main themes, points, headings that you started with, leaving them with a final summary of your talk.

They go away with the main themes clear in their minds.

In doing this, your listeners have received the same information three times, by way of the introduction, by you expanding on these themes in the main part of your talk, and by summarising things at the end.

And we know that repeating your exposure to information, particularly when there is some overall structure, where the info relates to a number of clear themes or ideas, and ideally where the information is personally relevant to you or you can imagine how you might use the information in practice, makes that information much more memorable.

So how does this relate to talking to your Reiki students as you progress through their course?

How to make your Reiki course content memorable

Well, you can explain to begin with what is going to be happening during their day, the big items, the main themes or headings.

Tell them what they are going to learning about and practising in the morning, and what they will do in the afternoon. I know they will have seen your course schedule in advance but it's a good idea to remind them on the day.

Then, whether you're giving people a quick talk about 'What Reiki is and where it comes from' or 'What Reiki can do for you and the people around you', or whether you are introducing Hatsurei ho or explaining about scanning, you can follow the "tell them, tell them, tell them" sequence: outline the main points, expand on them and then summarise.

Outline, expand, summarise.

Then move on to the next chunk of your day.

Recapping after a break

When you have had a break (your mid-morning break or the lunch break) it is very useful to give them a quick reminder of what they did earlier, summarise the main points very briefly and then move on to the next section, but showing how the next chunk of your day relates to

31

what has come before: how it follows on, how it builds on what they have already done.

You might use a phrase like:

"before the break what we did was to…"

"we learned that.…"

"and you discovered that…"

"now we are going to move on by learning about… and practising…"

If you taught Hatsurei ho and had a break, and now you are going to go through self-treatments, you might end up saying something like this (off the top of my head):

"So, before the break we went through Hatsurei ho, a set of daily energy exercises that you can use every day to start to balance your energy system: to clear, cleanse and ground you.

"You started by using Kenyoku – the dry bathing – where you ritually cleared and cleansed your energy system and then you moved on to move the energy to and from your tanden in time with your breathing, finally focusing the energy on your hands.

"It doesn't take too long to do, is a wonderful exercise to get into the habit of doing, and the audio CD that came in your study pack talks you through all the stages, so you can relax and just follow the instructions.

"Now we're going to move on to learn how to carry out a self-treatment. There are lots of different ways of doing self-treatments, most of them involving resting your hands on different parts of the body and letting the energy flow.

"Basically you are firing the energy from lots of different directions to give it the best chance to get to where it needs to go.

"But sometimes people can find the hand positions a bit awkward or uncomfortable to hold for any amount of time, so fortunately from original Japanese Reiki comes a self-treatment method actually taught by Mikao Usui, where you imagine that the energy is focusing on different areas of your head, and that's what we are going to go through.

"By treating the head, you actually end up treating the whole body anyway, and it's a lovely routine that you can go through whenever you have the opportunity to close your eyes for a few minutes.

"So, this is what we do…"

PS.

Please do not do this…

As an aside I wanted to say that you should never read a book or manual out loud to your students.

- It is unprofessional.
- It's so boring: not everyone reads out loud well.
- They can read it themselves so they don't need you to do it for them.

I have heard of courses where most of what happened was the teacher reading out loud to the student from a manual.

This is disgraceful behaviour!

They are there to learn from *you*, not to hear how well you can read out someone else's book.

Never read stuff out to students.

You may as well be a performing parrot.

Reiki teaching: using learning preferences

People learn in different ways. When we learn we take in information through our senses, so we see things, we hear things, we learn through doing and we mull things over in our mind. The best learning comes when you provide people with training that engages with all these aspects.

Some people tend to prefer one approach over the others, so you might find that one person much prefers to listen, whereas another might really need to see something before they 'get it', while yet others need to do practical things, to move, to really understand and remember what they are being presented with.

In NLP (Neurolinguistic Programming) these preferences are called being visual, or auditory or kinaesthetic. There is another preference, too, when people are referred to as 'audio digital': these people need a strong sense of order or logic before things sink in properly for them.

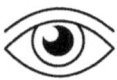 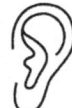 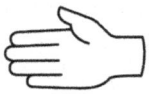 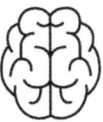

I am quite a visual person, so I like diagrams, I think in pictures (not everyone does), I use Mind Maps, my written notes are quite visually diverse and sometimes flamboyant.

I need that visual input more than, say, listening to something. And I have a great need for logic and order.

"The SatNav episode"

This was brought home to me several years ago when I was training in NLP and my wife Lorraine and I were going somewhere fairly local that we had not been to before.

We had the SatNav on but hadn't bothered to attach it to the windscreen; Lorraine had it resting in her lap and she looked at it and told me where to go.

Lorraine prefers the auditory sense so it made sense to her to just call out the instructions to me on this fiddly route; she said that I didn't need to see the screen. I thought that I didn't… But I did! I really did!

It was excruciating for me to travel without seeing a map of where I was going.

I had to stop the car in the end and look at the SatNav screen so I could *see* where I was. Once I had seen the territory it all made sense and I understood where I needed to go.

I needed to see to understand, whereas Lorraine didn't have that need.

When I give directions to someone I always want to reach for a scrap of paper so I can show someone; they might respond, though, by saying "just tell me!" My mind will be saying, "it's much better if I can show you."

But for them it may not be...

Don't assume everyone is just like you

The problem comes because we tend to assume that the way we learn is they way that everybody learns.

So if you learn by listening, you might run a course where you spend most of your time talking, and there will be students who are desperate to see something demonstrated, or to see a diagram, or to have an overview of what they day will entail, or to see the logical links between things, or to try something out for themselves, to 'get their hands dirty'.

So by running a course where you show things, you talk about things, you supervise people practising stuff, and you make sure that your day flows logically from one thing to another, you are providing your students with the very best training.

You are touching all bases and making sure that the course meets the learning preferences of all your students.

And by touching all bases, you actually make the learning more meaningful and effective for everyone, because the best learning uses sights, sounds and physicality, no matter what someone's preference might be. So a 'visual' learner like me needs images, but I will learn better if I also get to hear and to do.

Make your courses touch all bases

- On a live course it is straightforward to make sure that you are touching all bases: On a First Degree course, for example:
- Talk to them about Reiki and about the exercises they will be carrying out
- Show them what they will be doing when they perform the movements of Hatsurei ho and a Self-treatment
- Have them go through the physical movements with you
- Make sure they have seen you make the movements and practised the physical movements for themselves before they close their eyes for you to guide them with your voice

When dealing with the subject of treating other people, you can talk about the subject and then you can give a visual demonstration of the hand positions, talking to your students when you do that to give hints and tips and useful advice.

They then go through the hand positions themselves, guided by your voice.

Teaching materials to use on the day

You might consider having some display boards set up, with colour photographs demonstrating full treatment hand positions. Your students will take the information in subconsciously during the day.

On my Reiki Master Teacher live courses I used to have display boards set up which showed the stages of giving Western-style attunements.

They can see the visuals as you talk them through the process, then you give them a visual demonstration, then they go through the movements themselves with you or another student talking them through the stages.

I even had some A3 sheets and marker pens so students could draw little diagrams to explain the attunement stages, and I also had students sit down and talk each other through the process.

So I was engaging with all senses: they looked and were were watching, they listened and they explained; it is very powerful having someone explain something to another person because you have to have things well-ordered in your mind in order to do that.

They created visuals and they carried out physical movements while receiving spoken instructions.

All in all, a powerful learning combination.

Create materials that engage all senses

At Reiki Evolution we use detailed and comprehensive course manuals containing text, summaries and photographs.

The manuals are well ordered and logical and students get to read about the experiences of many other students that have been through this training.

Along with the printed manual, students for First Degree also receive separate "at a glance" summary sheets with lots of photographs to illustrate the stages of carrying out Hatsurei ho, giving a Self-treatment, and some Full treatment hand positions.

I include some blank 'cartoon strip'-style squares for them to do little drawings, perhaps just with stick figures, to illustrate the treatment hand positions, to jog their memory.

I also include a set of "20 Reiki questions", the answers to which they are expected to search for in their course materials, and I include a separate sheet with the answers that they can look at to check their discoveries.

We provide audio CDs with commentary (just like listening to a Reiki training course, but something that you can play again and again) and we also provide guided meditations, talking students through their daily energy exercises, a self-treatment meditation, a distant healing meditation and a Reiki symbol meditation.

You can see why we do that, can't you?

We provide logic and order, we provide written information, summaries and images, we provide short talks you can listen to and we give you the chance to be guided as you put Reiki into practice on yourself and with other people.

Engaging with people's different learning preferences, and ensuring that your live course and your training materials are multimedia, leads to the most powerful and effective learning.

Reiki teaching: using the right 4MAT

That is not a spelling mistake: I did intend to spell the word 'format' in that way! The "4MAT" system is a way of approaching teaching that was created by Bernice McCarthy and proposes that there are four major learning styles, each of which result in a student asking different questions and displaying different strengths during the learning process.

The 4MAT system is based on Myers-Briggs personality typing, which break people down into different categories, for example Introvert and Extrovert.

I am not going to go into detail here about the different categories (you can read up about those for yourself if you're interested) but beyond Introvert/Extrovert there are three other pairs of categories:

- Sensor/Intuitor
- Thinker/Feeler
- Judger/Perceiver

Myers Briggs uses these labels to create four-letter abbreviations for particular personality types, so someone might be an "INFJ", an Introvert, Intuitor,

Feeler, Judger. Myers Briggs aficionados will know immediately what sort of a person that is!

But let's get back to teaching and Reiki...

The four 4MAT categories

The 4MAT system describes four different types of learners, all of whom require different things in order to best assimilate information. Here are the four types:

The Concrete-Random learner

This learner needs to know "**Why?**" they are learning a particular thing, why they should be involved in a particular activity. What is the point of all this?

The Abstract-Sequential learner

This learner needs to know "**What?**" to learn: exactly what do they need to know? They need to see it in black and white; it shouldn't be vague and wishy-washy. There shouldn't be unanswered questions.

The Concrete-Sequential learner

This learner wants to know "**How?**" to apply the information they are being presented with: what do you actually do with this information in practice?

The Abstract-Random learner

This learner wants to answer "**What If?**" questions about how they can modify what they have learned to make it work for them.

Using 4MAT in practice

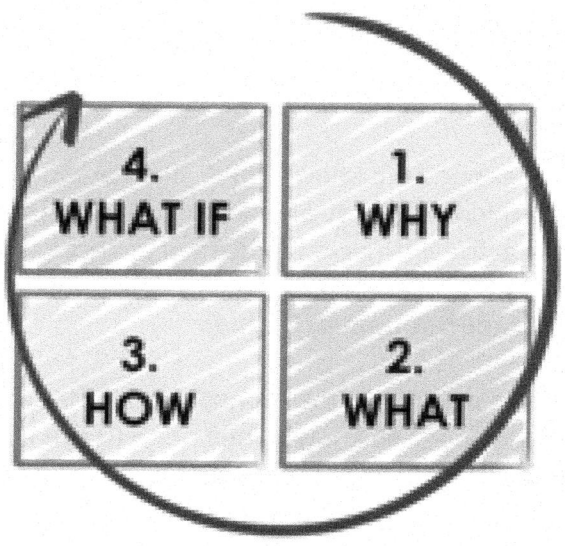

You can use the four questions – Why?, What?, How? and What If? to guide you when teaching a course or teaching a particular technique or practice.

If you deal with these four different questions, you make the learning accessible to the four major categories of learners, make what you teach memorable and ensure that you leave no-one behind.

These four questions can be cycled through again and again for each section of your course.

Let's think of an example: say, the teaching of Hatsurei ho (daily energy exercises used in Japanese-style Reiki). This is how the teaching of it, 4MAT-style, might look like:

Teach "Hatsurei ho" 4MAT-style

Why do we do Hatsurei ho? What is the purpose of it and what are our goals in carrying it out?

You can talk about how Hatsurei ho is a series of energy exercises that you carry out daily to clear and cleanse your energy system, ground you, and build up your ability as a channel over time.

What do we actually do when we perform Hatsurei ho? What are the stages, what precisely will we do in what order? What do we need to know in order to perform Hatsurei ho effectively?

You can talk about the individual stages, what you will be doing with your hands, what you will be imagining, how you tie in visualisation and the movement of energy with your breath.

How do we do Hatsurei ho? This would be a good time to talk your students through the process and talk about when to do Hatsurei ho, how often, and what happens if you miss a day.

Finally, how can you modify Hatsurei ho and use it in different contexts? This is the "**What If**?" stage: you might talk about separating out Kenyoku and using it for cleansing/clearing prior to starting a Reiki treatment, or in other situations.

You might also talk about using just Kenyoku and Joshin Kokkyu ho, a shorter sequence which comes closer to what Usui Sensei was teaching to his students in Japan.

That's not a bad sequence to keep cycling through, is it?

Teach "Scanning" 4MAT-style

Let's look at another example - "Scanning", - and how the 4MAT system helps us to teach this practice:

Why do we do use Scanning? What is the purpose of it and what are our goals in carrying it out?

You can talk about how scanning is a good way of 'getting the lie of the land' before you treat someone, finding out where the areas are that you're likely to be spending longer treating, that it is a good way of getting into the 'Reiki' state of mind, connecting with the energy, getting the energy flowing nicely before you start the treatment proper, and a way of building up your sensitivity to the energy through regular practice.

What do we actually do when we scan?

You can talk about the way that you hover your hands or hand over the body, how you focus your attention on the sensations that you can experience in your fingers and palm, and how you can drift from one area to another, going back and forth to check and double-check to see if you get a repeated 'spike' in sensations over a particular area.

What do we need to know in order to do scanning effectively?

How do we do scanning? This would be a good time to demonstrate and to talk your students through the process for real: guiding their movements, asking questions and commenting on what they notice, and making helpful suggestions.

Finally, you can deal with "**What If**?" questions: what if you can't feel anything in your hands, what if it all feels the same, what does it mean if you notice a particular sensation, like heat, or fizzing, or coldness, or a breeze, or pulsing? How else do Reiki people use scanning?

In both these examples, you introduce a topic or exercise by explaining why you would want to go through this exercise, you move on to explain in detail exactly what the exercise is, you describe how the exercise is used or carried out in practice and then finish by exploring different ways in which the exercise can be used, in different contexts and situations, and deal with common questions that people have.

So you can see that the 4MAT system provides you with a way of being comprehensive with your teaching of each chunk of your course, while meeting the learning needs of all your students.

Over to you

Why not look at the different things that you teach on your Reiki courses, and see how well your presentations, descriptions and demonstrations meet these four learning criteria.

How could you alter what you say and do to follow the 4MAT system in these examples?

- Self-treatments
- Head/shoulder treatments
- Distant healing
- Using the Reiki symbols
- Working intuitively

Reiki teaching: your course materials

Imagine going on a Reiki course, say a First Degree course, for the first time. You don't know anything about Reiki, really, and you're not sure what is going to happen on the course.

When you arrive, the teacher starts to tell you huge amounts of information about Reiki during your day. It's difficult to take it all in – it's all so new, after all, and you haven't heard any of this stuff before.

There are new ideas and concept to get your head around and you have lots of questions.

You try to take notes as you go along, but it's a bit like trying to drink from a fire hose. You scribble away, and while you're concentrating on what to write down you miss the next bit of what they are saying, and you can hardly replay what they just said!

The attunements or empowerments you receive, while often wonderful experiences, don't help either because they have made you feel all spaced out and blissful, and the energy work is zonking you out too, as you try and concentrate on what is being said.

There's a lot to take in.

Then, at the end of the day, you get sent home with a cheery goodbye and two sheets of A4: one with your lineage and one with a bad photocopy of some treatment hand positions.

Reiki students deserve better than that.

So what I am going to talk about in this article are two things that you can do to make sure that your students' experience does not match what I described above.

You can:

- Provide extensive course materials
- Send out course materials to students in advance

Provide extensive course materials

Your students need to relax, safe in the knowledge that everything you say on their Reiki course is covered in detail in their course materials.

You should lay out everything that you teach, clearly and logically, with summaries, illustrations or images, and expand on what you teach on the day, providing non-essential but useful information that rounds out and deepens their knowledge of the system that they are learning.

Your students should not be forced to take notes because this is a huge distraction, stops them from enjoying the day, and trying to take decent notes when you're all zonked out on energy is no fun.

So your students deserve a proper course manual that covers *everything* that you dealt with on the course, with further explanations, examples, and back-up info.

They should be able to use your manual as a reference work that they can return to again and again to check on everything that is needed for that level.

Give your students variations to experiment with: there is no 'one true way' with Reiki, so suggest different self-treatment methods, and show how they can treat people in different ways, for example short blasts on someone's sore back at work, say, head/shoulder treatments, and full treatments.

Cover everything that you say on a live course, absolutely everything, and more besides, and deal with every question that a student has asked you so that what you provide is really comprehensive: a valuable long-term resource.

Your course materials will be a 'work-in-progress' for some time!

You should also deal with students' learning preferences and make your materials multimedia, and I will talk about this more in a later article.

Send you materials out in advance

Many years ago when I first started teaching Reiki, I was talking to a Reiki Master that I met at a Reiki gathering or meeting and she mentioned to me that she always sent her students a Reiki manual in advance, before they arrived on the day of their course.

My first reaction, because it was different to how I had been taught, was to think, "no, no, no, that's all wrong!" but it didn't take very long before I realised that, actually, that was a genius idea. I wish I could remember her name so I could thank her!

By sending a Reiki manual as soon as a student books on their course, they can take their time and read about Reiki, what it is and where it comes from, what it can do for them, how it can help people you treat, at their leisure.

There is no reason why all this information has to be blasted at a student for the first time on the day of a course.

They can mull over the information, think about it, search for answers to any questions that they might have, reflect on what they have read.

They will also read about the practical exercises that they are going to be guided through on their live course, so they will already be fairly familiar with Hatsurei ho (daily energy exercises), self-treatments and treating others in different ways.

Info is better assimilated over time, in manageable chunks, rather than trying to 'drink from a fire hose' on the day of a course.

In fact, when I send out study packs to my Reiki Evolution students, I include a couple of audio CDs, a sheet where they can note down their Reiki goals and their initial questions, and I also give them a list of 20 questions that they should be able to answer.

I do this so that their subconscious is primed to look for those answers in the course materials, and once they have found the answers then they have focused on the main points or areas that I wanted them to focus on.

By doing this, when they arrive on their live course they are already quite clued-up about Reiki and what they are going to be doing on their live course:

1. The teacher does not have to spend their time sitting down telling the students stuff that they could have easily read about beforehand
2. Students can spend most of their time on the live course actually doing stuff with energy rather than sitting hearing someone talk about, say, the history of Reiki
3. The teacher can spend their time just recapping what the students are already familiar with, focusing the students on the main points and themes and thus reinforcing them

If you're on a live course, it makes sense to make the time you spend count, to make it mostly about experiencing energy and practising using energy on yourself and on other people, rather than just sitting telling students stuff.

Reiki is a practical skill, after all, and rather like riding on a bicycle, you should spend your time practising it, not hearing about it!

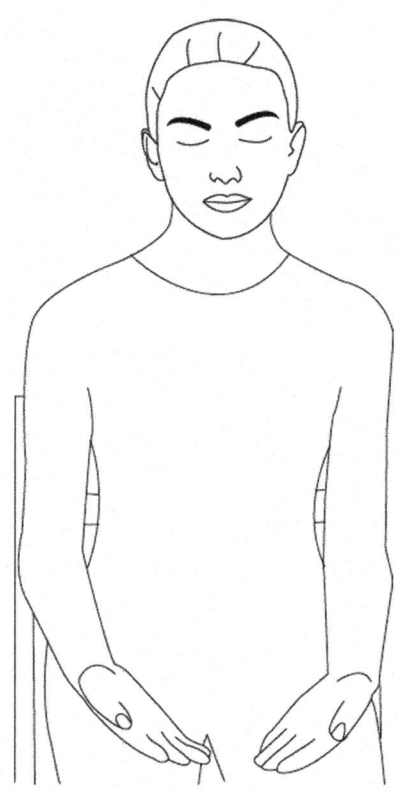

Reiki teaching: How to create your Reiki manual

Your students need to relax, safe in the knowledge that everything you say on their Reiki course is covered in detail in their course materials.

You should lay out everything that you teach, clearly and logically, with summaries, illustrations or images, and expand on what you teach on the day, providing non-essential but useful information that rounds out and deepens their knowledge of the system that they are learning.

Your students should not be forced to take notes because this is a huge distraction, stops them from enjoying the day, and trying to take decent notes when you're all zonked out on energy is no fun.

So your students deserve a proper course manual that covers *everything* that you dealt with on the course, with further explanations, examples, and back-up info.

They should be able to use your manual as a reference work that they can return to again and again to check on everything that is needed for that level.

You start with your notes

Your Reiki manual should start with what you tell students on their live course, so at the very least they have a hard copy of everything that you say to them, to refer to after their course. They won't be able to remember, or take notes on, everything that you said to them, after all.

So you can base your manual on the notes that you made when you put your live course together.

Write down everything that you think you say to people during your course and that can give you a basic lot of content to work with.

And because your notes will follow the basic order of your course, your manual will also follow that logical structure, which is helpful.

But when you teach, live, you will probably say more than you just jotted down in your notes: you will probably expand on things, give different real-world examples of people that you have treated, for example, to illustrate different points. I would hazard a guess that all of that won't be there in your notes.

But all these things need to go in your manual, too, to make sure that it is comprehensive and detailed: a true resource for your students to be able to refer to and rely on. So how do you make that happen?

Record yourself when you teach

Use a hand-held audio recorder to record yourself during your courses. Simple recorders can be picked up cheaply, they record and play back, and many have an integral usb plug so you can plug them straight into your PC or laptop and drag and drop the audio tracks for listening later.

You may not like listening to the sound of your voice but (a lot of people don't) but you just need to get over yourself and do it anyway, to be honest with you, because your manual will be so much more useful as a result.

Anything that you explain on a course, that you haven't already noted down, you should write down now: all the anecdotes, all the explanations, all the descriptions and helpful practical suggestions that you make: add all of these to your manual.

But when we teach Reiki, often new topics of conversation arise.

Students come up with so many different questions that you hadn't prepared for and for which there are no answers in your notes: you have to deal with queries and issues 'on the fly', using your knowledge and experience there and then to help your students to be clear about what they should do.

This is a very useful resource for you.

Use students' questions to guide you

Can you remember what interesting question or questions someone asked you the last time you taught Reiki? Maybe you made a note of them somewhere.

Questions asked by your students are an absolute goldmine of useful content for your course materials!

You can put those answers or that issue in your manual to make sure that if anyone else wondered about that topic, you already have it covered.

Because, of course, if one person has asked that question, you can be sure that many other students will be thinking about, and wondering about, the same thing, whether or not they ask about it out loud.

Think back on other courses you held (or even courses that you attended when you were learning Reiki) and see if you can remember what interesting points and issues came up.

All these issues can go in your manual.

But maybe you haven't taught any Reiki courses yet; maybe you are getting your manual together in advance, ready for your first course or courses.

That's ok, because your manual should not be set in stone…

Make your manual a work in progress

Your Reiki manual does not have to be set in stone, a once-in-a-lifetime achievement that is never altered or changed once you have completed it.

It would be more useful for you to see it as a work in progress: a manual that is 'good enough', but not there quite yet.

So as you carry on teaching Reiki, and have to deal with further interesting questions and queries, or areas where people seem confused or need further explanations to really 'get it', you can put all those explanations in your manual, adding to it every few weeks.

Over time, you will answer more and more of your students' questions, each time making your manual more and more comprehensive and useful.

You will create a valuable resource that your students can go back to again and again, each time discovering something new or different that supports them no matter where they are on their journey with Reiki.

And while we're talking about making your manual useful, there is something that you can do that will really help your students, which is to...

Give your students options and choices

Now, there is no 'one true way' when it comes to Reiki, so it is helpful and empowering to suggest different ways that people can carry out a meditation or a self-treatment or give a treatment to someone else.

If you do that, you can encourage your students to experiment and find out for themselves what works best for them.

This is a good thing because you are allowing them to develop some flexibility in their approach and giving them ownership of the process.

So explain to them various self-treatment methods, and show how they can treat others in different ways, for example: short blasts on someone's sore back at work, head/shoulder treatments on someone sitting in a chair, and full treatments on someone lying on a treatment couch.

Explain how they can take Kenyoku out of Hatsurei ho and use it whenever they like, during their day or before giving a hands-on treatment.

Talk about how some people use scanning as a way of feeling the quality of the energy emanating from various foodstuffs in the supermarket, to help them decide which items would be best for them to buy.

Share these things as options, even if you do not practise them yourself.

Use anecdotes, case studies and testimonials

The most powerful way to illustrate and emphasise the main points that you want to get across to your students is to use stories about real people that you have worked with – either whom you have treated or whom you have taught.

So if you are talking about the effects that Reiki can have on people who receive a course of Reiki treatments, illustrate this by talking about the experiences of some of the people that you have treated.

You don't need to identify them by name, but you could say that you treated a lady once who had a problem x and this is what happened.

If one of your clients has given you a testimonial to use, where they talk about what their problem was and how Reiki helped them, you could use that, too, by way of backing up what you are saying.

If you are talking about how being attuned to Reiki can often bring things to the surface to be released, giving students a bit of a rough ride for a while, you could talk about the experiences of someone you have taught, or quote some feedback that they sent you, where they talk about their 'Reiki cold' or their emotional ups and downs etc, or where they talk about their sudden desire to de-clutter their house or simplify their life..

Reiki teaching: How to create a Reiki Audio CD

You may feel daunted enough at the prospect of putting together a good quality Reiki manual, so that the whole idea of recording an hour's worth of audio commentary fills you with dread, and I can understand that.

Certainly I was daunted at the whole idea.

Partly this was because I felt rather self-conscious about the way that my voice sounds and didn't like hearing recordings of me speaking, so the idea of students listening to my voice wasn't appealing.

Secondly, it occurred to me that, unlike when you talk to students on a live Reiki course, where when you say something it's then gone, lost, never to be listened to again… with an audio recording that a student will be listening to, you do need to get it right.

I was intimidated at the prospect of crafting what I thought needed to be the perfect representation of an idea or phrase.

But we are getting a little ahead of ourselves…

Find your voice

My advice to you would be to not create an audio CD, or audio programme on MP3, until you have been teaching Reiki courses for a while.

You need to be comfortable with the format and content of your courses and you need to have found your own comfortable way of talking about Reiki, explaining things and guiding students through practical exercises and meditations in your own words.

Only when you have 'found your voice' should you think about recording audio tracks, so that your carefully-crafted phrases – which you have used repeatedly on your live courses - almost 'trip off your tongue'.

You need to be comfortable and familiar with what you are going to be saying.

Find your content

In my article on creating your own Reiki manual, I suggested that a good place to start would be to record yourself when you talk to people on your live courses, and I recommend this again here.

When you explain things to students on the day of a course, assuming you don't have a tendency to fly off at a tangent and talk about irrelevancies, you will be explaining the main points, the main themes, the essential 'bullet points' of what you want to get across.

What you say to students on your course forms the backbone of what they should hear on their audio CD because the CD is there to provide students with your essential message, the principles and advice they you believe they should definitely remember and take away with them in order to practise Reiki effectively.

Your manual is based on the way that you structure your course, your audio CD is based on the way that you structure your course, so each chapter will have its own audio track.

Track listing from Reiki First Degree CD

I thought you might find it helpful to see the track listing from my First Degree audio CD and how long I spent talking about the various topics I decided on (minutes):

01	Introduction	2.45m
02	What is Reiki?	5.41m
03	Where did Reiki come from?	6.19m
04	What learning Reiki can do for you	4.32m
05	Following the original system	4.12m
06	The precepts and mindfulness	5.22m
07	The 5 precepts in Japanese	0.17m
08	Reiju empowerments	6.25m
09	Daily energy exercises	6.22m
10	Self-treatment approaches	6.35m
11	Giving and receiving treatments	7.10m
12	Different treatment approaches	4.09m
13	Full treatments: starting & scanning	6.29m
14	Full treatments: rest of treatment	4.13m

Avoid an excruciating experience

You will probably have listened to someone reading out a speech from their notes. It is just awful, isn't it? It can sound monotonous and uninteresting, with no light and shade, no emphasis and no colour.

You don't want to inflict that on your students.

So how do you make sure that you say what's important without fluffing your lines, while at the same time sounding like a human being?

Do this: write in the way that you talk.

Listen to recordings of you explaining things to students, in your own words, and write that down! Don't write a lecture: write down your own words in the way that comes naturally to you.

That's "Important advice part 1" of how to come across as natural and interesting.

"Important advice part 2" is to have your notes in front of you when you make your recording, but make sure that you have practised and rehearsed so many times that all the phrases are comfortable and familiar to you.

Make sure that you don't have to keep your eyes on your notes at all times: be sufficiently familiar with what you are going to say that the notes are just there to act as a reminder, not something where you have to cling onto every written word for fear of forgetting.

Practise. Then practise some more. Come back to it another day. Practise some more.

Then you're ready to record.

The nuts and bolts of what to do

It's beyond the scope of this book to give you detailed advice about audio recording and editing, but you'd be surprised by how straightforward it is.

To record yourself you could use the 'record' function on your smart phone, you could use an inexpensive hand-held voice recorder, or you could use a microphone plugged into your laptop or PC.

If using a microphone, you can choose between a 'Lavalier' clip-onto-your-lapel condenser mic, a 'boom mic', or a table-mounted microphone.

I recommend the Blue Yeti USB microphone but I have had good results with a boom mic too.

For audio editing, if you have an Apple product it will come with Garageband, or for all computer users (Macs included) you can use "Audacity", which is a free, open-source piece of audio editing software which is simple to use and for which there are endless 'how to…' videos on YouTube. I recommend Audacity.

Once you have your collection of tracks, you can burn them to a CD-R or have them printed professionally.

A few Audacity tips

Audacity will export recordings as WAV files (which you burn onto a CD to create an audio CD that will play on CD players (or computers), and it will also create MP3s for you if you have also installed the LAME encoder (which is easier than it sounds)!

Start each recording with, say, ten seconds of silence (background noise) so that you have something to sample when you come to the stage of noise reduction, and remember to 'normalise' each track before you export them.

Edit the tracks so that there are a couple of seconds of silence at the beginning and end of the tracks, and they can then be exported in WAV or MP3 format.

The 'noise reduction' function listens to a representative sample of background noise and uses that as the basis for its noise reduction efforts on your track; this function works well.

To explain 'normalise', do you remember when you made 'mix tapes' or burned 'compilation CDs' and sometimes you found that some of the tracks seemed louder or quieter than the others (so you had to turn the volume up, or rush to turn the volume down) when you played the compilation cassette/CD?

That was because the different source tapes/CDs had been recorded at different volume levels.

The way to make sure that all your audio tracks are playing at the same volume level, you need to 'normalise' them, and this compensates for your voice perhaps being a bit louder or quieter on different tracks.

It's easy to do because you just highlight the track and hit 'Normalise'!

These comments will make perfect sense once you have started using the software for yourself, looked at instructional videos on YouTube and after you have Googled such topics as:

- "how to normalise a track in Audacity"
- "why should I normalise a track in Audacity
- "how to do noise reduction using Audacity"
- "how to install LAME encoder Audacity"

How to use your CD in practice

When you send your students their study pack in advance, which is what I recommend, they can use their audio CD and their course manual in combination with each other.

What they can do is this, for each section of their manual:

1. Listen to the track that relates to the chapter in their manual, which gives them a good overview of that topic
2. Read the chapter in your manual, which adds extra details and expands their knowledge

3. Listen to the audio track again, to bring things back to the main themes they need to remember

You have thus gone through the:

- Tell them what you are going to tell them
- Tell them
- Tell them what you told them

…sequence that I mentioned earlier on: give them the basic theme, expand on that, and bring them back to the main points.

And by having a permanent record of your voice, they will be able to, in effect, listen to your Reiki course again and again: a day later, a week later, and months later.

Many people find that, in doing this, they notice different things on each playing, as their knowledge and experience progresses; they take what they need on each occasion.

Such benefits are missing entirely if they only got to hear you talking about a topic once, on the weekend of your Reiki course, when they were probably zonked out on the energy in any case, because of the empowerments or attunements you gave them!

Far better for them to be able to 'take their course home with them' and benefit from your wisdom at their leisure.

If you create an audio CD or a MP3 collection for your students, you will have created a really beneficial resource for them. I recommend it.

Reiki teaching: supporting your students

One of the things that we hear about quite a lot from people who come to Reiki Evolution, having taken a Reiki course before with a different teacher, is that they were never able to get in touch with their previous teacher to ask questions or ask for advice.

They felt left out on a limb.

Either the teacher never got back to them, or the student had the impression that the teacher was 'too busy', or the student felt intimidated and didn't want to 'bother' their Reiki teacher.

That's not very good, is it?

So in this article I thought I would talk a bit about the different ways that we can support our students.

Decent course materials and training

The first way that we can help our students to have a great Reiki experience is to make sure that we deal with the common questions that students ask, on our live courses and in our course materials.

When I first started to teach Reiki my students had a lot of questions, and what I did was to remember what a student had asked and make sure that I provided the answer to that question the next time I ran that course, so that over time my courses because more and more helpful, and my course materials because more and more comprehensive.

Over time, I found that the number of questions I received reduced because I was answering them all in advance!

Be happy to help

Make it clear to students that you are happy to answer any questions that they might have, once they have completed their training.

Have a state of mind of being friendly, open and supportive and your students will pick up on that.

I tell people that the only stupid question is the question that you do not ask, where you still have this need to have something explained to you, running round your head. That would be the stupid thing!

Now that does not mean that you have to be the source of all Reiki knowledge, on tap, available 24/7. You don't want students asking you questions that are right there in their manual.

You can refer them to sources of information, like sections of your manual, or blog posts that you have written, or give them links to web sites etc.

And not all questions are answerable anyway, or the answer might be "who knows?" or "who knows, and it doesn't really matter anyway"

Remember that you are not the source of all Reiki wisdom that your students need to consult for answers about everything: we should not encourage students to be dependent on us as teachers.

You initiate them and they set out on their own journey of discovery and experimentation.

But having said that, you should do what you can to point them in the right direction and keep them focused on the important aspects of Reiki.

Reiki shares

At their most basic, Reiki shares are Reiki get-togethers where you meet other Reiki people and swap Reiki treatments. If there are a fair number of people attending, everyone takes a turn on the treatment table and can end up being treated by multiple practitioners: you might have one person sitting at the head of the table, someone by your ankles and people on either side of the table too.

Receiving a Reiki treatments from lots of people at the same time is an *amazing* experience!

Highly recommended.

Sometimes the Reiki share host (it doesn't have to be a Reiki Master but often is) will talk people though some energy exercises (for example kanyoku followed by Joshin Kokkyu ho) and give attunements (or ideally Reiju empowerments) to everyone present.

If there are several Reiki Masters present, they could 'share out' the empowerments and do a few each. This is ideal if there are new Reiki Masters there who want to practise giving empowerments to people.

Sometimes there might be a further guided meditation or a group distant healing session or a chat about people's experiences when treating other people, say.

You can do what you like.

Set a particular date, say the first Thursday in the month at 7.30pm, or the second Saturday at 2pm, and see what happens.

Reiki practice days

This is a variation on a Reiki share where people have the opportunity to give and receive full Reiki treatments, in pairs, while under the supervision of a Reiki teacher, and is ideal for people who have taken a First Degree course, say, and who haven't had too much of a chance to treat other people, or people who learned Reiki some time ago and now want to get going properly and build their confidence.

The day could again start with some energy exercises and empowerments, and could include a question-and-answer session.

Online support networks

I am a great believer in students providing support to each other, rather than feeling that they have to be dependent on their teacher. Everyone has useful experience that they can share with each other. The Reiki teacher does not know everything, after all.

There are different ways of providing such support, some simpler than others, for example:

A Yahoo! Group

A NING site

A Facebook group

In all these examples, students are able to talk to each other, whether that is through swapping email messages with the whole group (Yahoo!), chatting one-to-one or posting videos and images.

Groups like this can build a tremendous sense of community and you can be sure that if one person posts a question, there will be many other students who were wondering about that too, but didn't ask!

People will share their successes, their amazement, their awe and enthusiasm and the interesting things that have happened to them and to the people they treated.

Some will talk about the changes the have noticed within themselves since starting to use Reiki regularly and how they precepts have altered the way they behave and feel about things and changed in the way respond to others.

Highly recommended.

And while to begin with, if you are just starting out as a teacher, you might only have a handful of students subscribed (and tumbleweed blowing through your chat rooms!) it won't be too long before the numbers build up and you'll have on hand a wealth of knowledge and experience that new students can draw upon.

How to run a Reiki share

What is a Reiki share?

At their most basic, Reiki shares are Reiki get-togethers where you meet other Reiki people and swap Reiki treatments.

If there are a fair number of people attending, everyone takes a turn on the treatment table and can end up being treated by multiple practitioners: you might have one person sitting at the head of the table, someone by your ankles and people on either side of the table too.

Why Reiki shares?

Receiving a Reiki treatments from lots of people at the same time is an *amazing* experience! If you have never experienced that, I really, really, really recommend that you find a Reiki share, jump on the table and see how it feels. You will be blown away!

It is also useful to spend some time in the company of people who do not think that you are crazy for doing this ridiculous energy thing, and you have the opportunity to share your experiences and ask questions.

For those who do not have many friends or family on hand to treat, Reiki shares can help to build your confidence and reassure you that all your 'Reiki apparatus' is working properly: you are more likely to receive useful feedback from a Reiki-attuned person being treated by you than you are a member of the general public.

And of course, for a Reiki Master, hosting a Reiki share is a very valuable service that you can provide to your most motivated students.

Do you need to be a Reiki Master to run a Reiki share?

Interestingly, no. Not at all. Anyone can set up and run a Reiki share. All you need are a small group of people willing to get together on a regular basis to swap Reiki treatments.

But if you are a Reiki Master, there is something that you will be able to do during your shares that wouldn't have been possible without a Reiki Master being present: giving people attunements or empowerments.

How popular are Reiki shares?

In my experience, although most Reiki people probably like the idea of Reiki shares, and would be disappointed to hear that one had discontinued, the vast majority of Reiki people will not have attended a Reiki share and probably never will.

That's just the way it is: people have busy lives, and it's always a very small minority of people that get actively involved in such things.

Having said that, all you really need is a small core of people who are prepared to make the time, perhaps just for one evening of afternoon a month, to get together with others to share Reiki, and you will have a successful share.

Where to hold a Reiki share

Many people hold Reiki shares in their own home. If participants are willing, you could take turns in different people's homes.

Perhaps you could use the venue where you run your Reiki courses, or you could hire a local hall, like a village hall. The venue does need to be warm enough to be comfortable on cold days, though.

Where to get treatment tables from

Since you're a Reiki Master Teacher you probably have a few treatment tables of your own that you can use.

Reiki practitioners will usually have their own table and even people who are not practising professionally may well have your own portable table: the participants can bring their tables with them.

You don't need loads of table, though: one table can accommodate 6-7 people taking turns at being treated.

What else do I need?

Blankets. Some people find that they can get a bit chilly while being treated, and being tucked up in a blanket can make the experience even more special.

A music player (e.g. a CD player or an iPod with a Bluetooth or other external speaker)

A clock or a wristwatch, or mobile phone that will display the time without turning black after a few minutes, or perhaps display a countdown timer (that does not have an alarm when it gets to zero!)

A way of having dimmed lights: Reiki shares aren't so pleasurable if you're lying underneath a big fluorescent light, so maybe bring a couple of lamps with you and turn the main lights off.

Refreshments. At the very least, people need to have some water available, but it would be nice for people to have a chance to sit down with a hot drink when they arrive, and while you are waiting for everyone to arrive.

Working out the timing

This is fairly straightforward, so if you have three people attending and you have allocated 90 minutes for the on-the-treatment-table sharing session, each person gets 25 minutes, with a break of five minutes for people to recover and have a drink of water.

If you have eight people using two treatment tables, with 90 minutes allocated to the treatments, there will be four people on each table.

Assume four breaks of 5 minutes each, so our 90 minutes have reduced to 70. 70 minutes shared amongst four people is about 18 minutes for each treatment.

Keeping track of time during the session

Whenever someone is being treated, one person will always sit at the head of the treatment table, working on the head and shoulders.

That person is responsible for keeping track of the time, usually by resting a wristwatch on the table so they can just glance at it occasionally.

A gentle way of letting everyone know that the session is over is, rather than saying, loudly, "right, time to stop now!", is to do this: breathe in deeply and then exhale loudly, while taking your hands off the recipient, rubbing your hands together as you move back away from the table.

This combination of moving and making the 'hand-rubbing' sound, and breathing out loudly, is usually enough to alert the other participants that the session is over, and you have achieved that in a gentle and unobtrusive way.

Where should people stand, around the treatment table?

This is not set in stone, but here are some useful combinations for different numbers of participants:

Three people

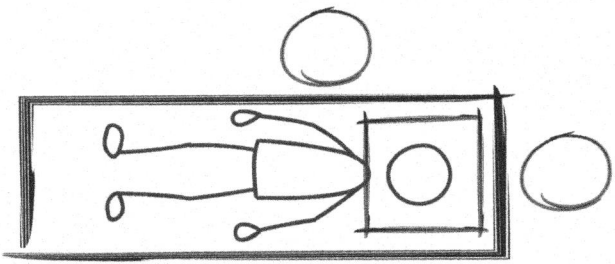

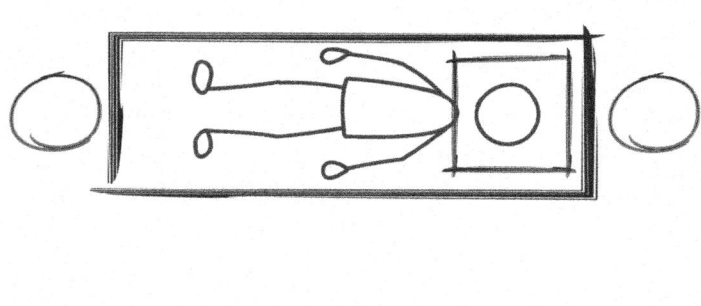

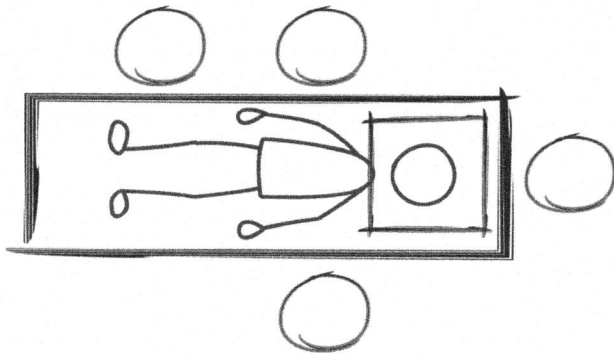

Four people

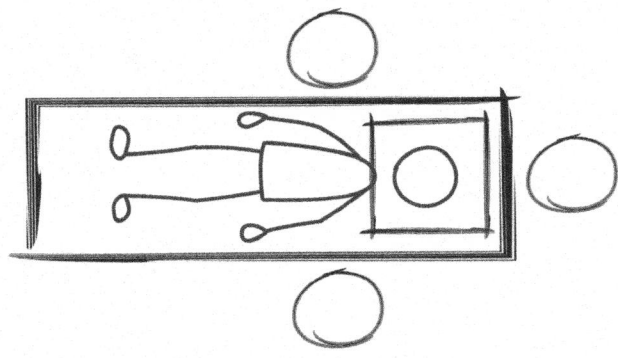

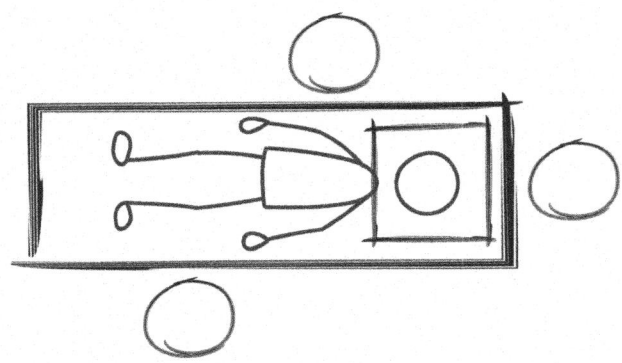

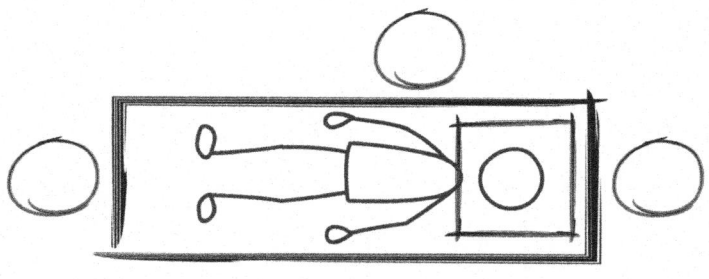

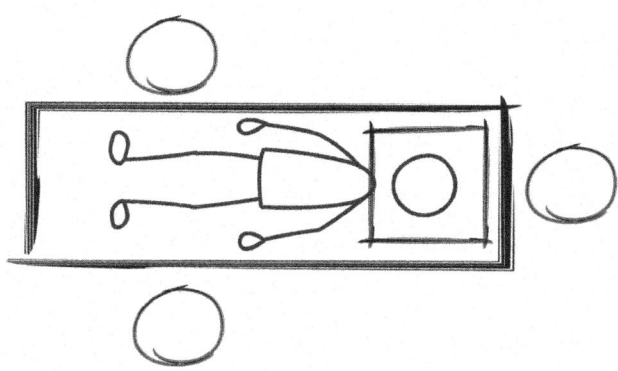

Five people

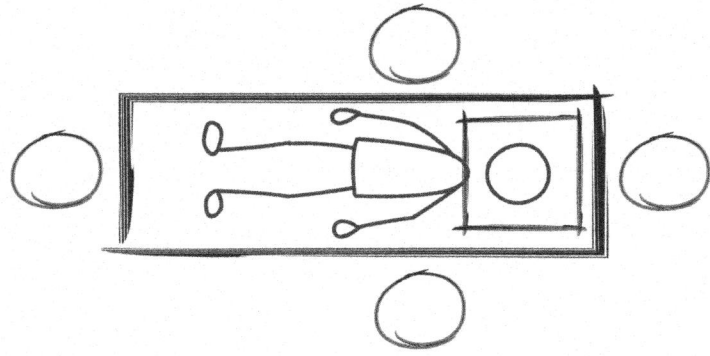

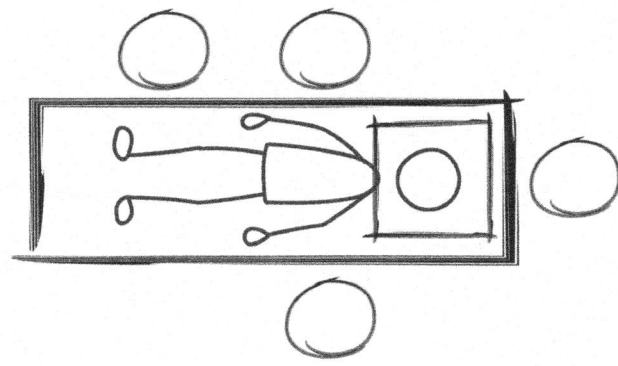

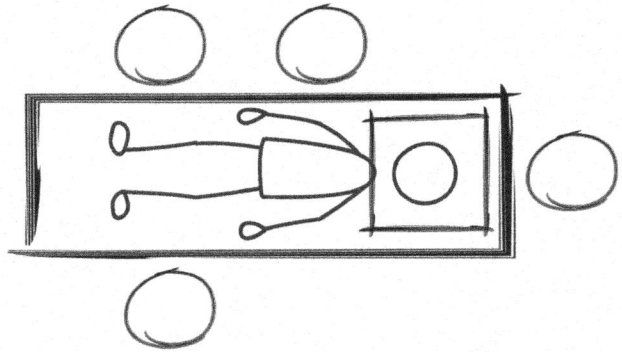

Six people

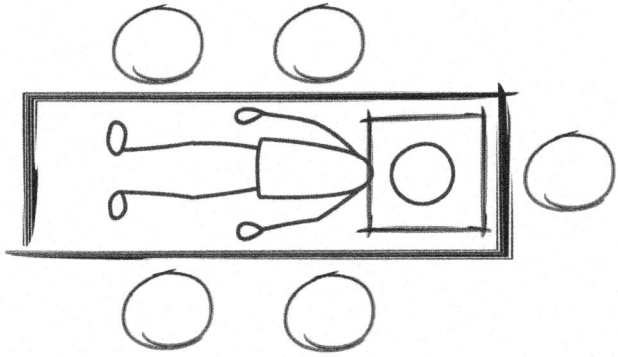

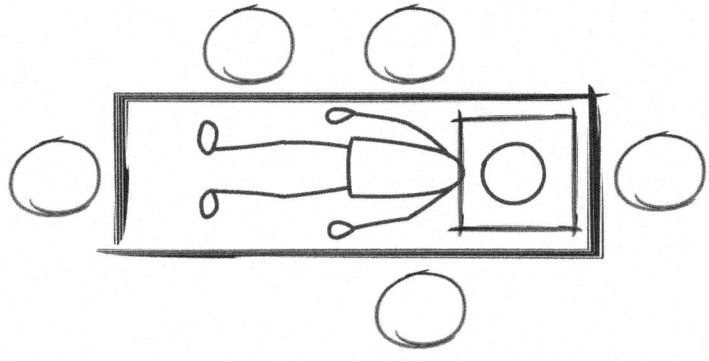

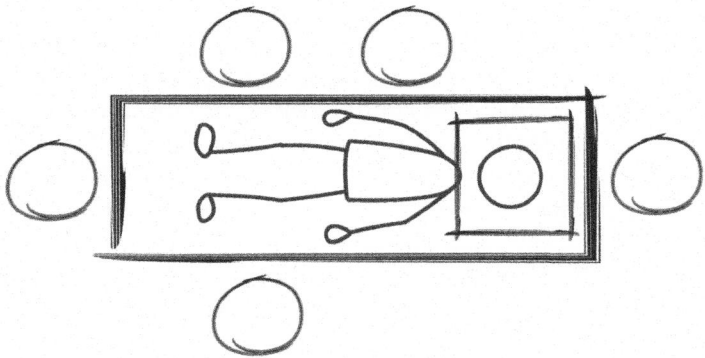

Seven people

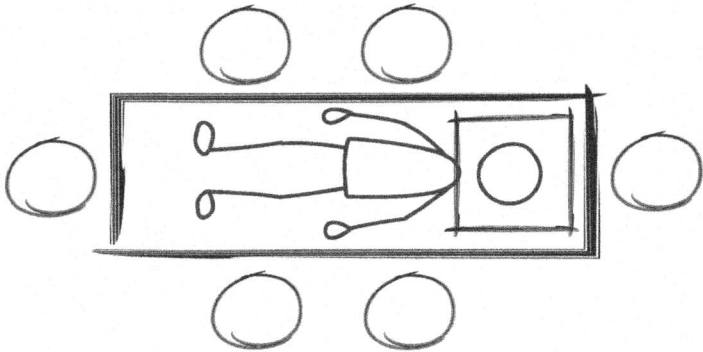

What hand positions should you use?

You can be really flexible with hand positions. They are not set in stone, as you know, and the person is going to be receiving Reiki that is channelled into them from lots of different places, so it does not really matter: it will be a wonderful experience for the recipient no matter where people put their hands!

If you're sitting at the head of the table, it would be nice to start by resting your hands on the shoulders for a few minutes.

Then you can use any of the hand positions that you already know; perhaps you will decide to cradle their head on your hands or perhaps you will decide to not disturb them, and stay off the body for the rest of the treatment.

If you are standing by the torso, you could rest one hand on the solar plexus and hover the other hand over the heart area (when treating a woman) or rest your hand on the heart area (when treating a man); all hand positions should be non-intrusive, of course.

You could then move on to treat both side of the abdomen (hands at the level of the navel) and treat both hips; you are constrained by the presence of other people giving the treatment, though, so if two of you are treating the torso, perhaps you could stay to your side, treating the abdomen and hip on your side of the body, perhaps while they do the same on the other side.

It can be powerful to mirror hand positions on either side of the midline.

Of course, if you are the only person standing on your side of the treatment table, you can range all the way along, almost from their shoulders to their ankles.

One area of the body that tends to get neglected during routine Reiki treatments is the arm, or the hand, and if you are standing by the torso then you could rest your hands on the recipient's elbow, and on their hand.

This can feel fantastic being on the receiving end, with a boiling hot 'Reiki hand' either resting on yours of holding your hand; lovely.

If you are standing by the legs, you will either be treating both sides of the body or just one side, depending on whether there is another Reiki person standing opposite you.

If you are on your own at the legs, you could treat both hips, both thighs, both knees and both ankles.

If there are two of you treating the legs, you could rest your hands on the hip and thigh, thigh and knee, or knee and ankle, or you might decide to cup your hands above and below the knee or the ankle.

If you are sitting at the foot of the treatment table – and it works better if you sit rather than stand – then you can spend a lot of time with your hands resting on the ankles, you might choose to lean forwards and rest your hands on the shins, or you might rest your palms against the soles of their feet; you might treat one foot and then the other, or work on both at the same time.

And whether or not anyone has been 'allocated' to the feet, it is nice for someone to move there at some stage during the session, or to end up there for a little while at the end of the session.

Finishing the treatment

It can be nice for someone to take responsibility for 'smoothing down the energy field' at the end of a session.

It's easier if this is someone who has been treating the torso or feet because they are already in the right sort of position; sometimes two people will do this in unison, on either side of the body, and that can be quite nice.

Using intuitively guided hand positions

For Reiki people who do not have too many opportunities to treat other people, a Reiki share can give them a chance to become comfortable with treating others, to receive positive feedback from the people they treated, and to have a chance to practise working intuitively on quite a few 'bodies'.

This can be very useful and build confidence quickly.

Other things to do at a Reiki share

Sometimes the Reiki share host will start things off by talking people though some energy exercises, for example Kenyoku followed by Joshin Kokkyu ho, just to get the energy flowing.

You could always talk people through the entire Hatsurei ho sequence if you liked.

Some people like to use the Reiki Evolution "Reiki Meditations" CD so that everyone can sit and be guided through the sequence together, and that works well.

Sometimes there might be a further guided meditation of some sort, or perhaps a group distant healing session or a chat about people's experiences when treating others, so the Reiki share can double as a sort of Practitioner support meeting.

You can do what you like.

Giving attunements or empowerments at a Reiki share

What works really well is to start the session by moving from Kenyoku/Joshin Kokkyu ho (or Hatsurei ho) straight into giving a Reiki initiation to everyone present.

Reiki attunements are often quite time-consuming and detailed, though, so it would be easier and quicker if people were to receive Reiju empowerments instead.

The effect is the same, of course, but people wouldn't have to sit there for potentially a very long time while the initiations are completed.

If there are several Reiki Masters present, they could 'share out' the empowerments and do a few each.

This is ideal if you have taught some people to Reiki Master Teacher level: these new Reiki Masters can practise giving empowerments to people, going through the movements in a nice, friendly, informal setting, without the pressure of having to 'get it right' because they are running a course.

How to run a Reiki practice day

What is a Reiki practice day?

This is I suppose a little bit like a Reiki share, where people have the opportunity to give and receive Reiki treatments, but they are doing this in pairs, or in groups of three, while under the supervision of a Reiki teacher.

So it is more of a follow-up teaching day, where students can get some more practice and have their questions answered.

It could be organised as a half-a-day for people at First Degree and a half-a-day for people at Second Degree, or you could mix both levels together.

Why run a Reiki practice day?

Reiki practice days are ideal for people who have taken a First Degree course and who haven't had too much of a chance to treat other people, so they're not feeling too confident yet and maybe they haven't received sufficient positive feedback from people they have worked on to feel that Reiki is definitely working for them.

Such a day is also ideally suited for people who have recently completed a Second Degree course and would like some supervised practice so they can explore the new approaches they were taught on their Second Degree course.

They can explore using intent, for example, practise opening to intuition, and they will receive probably more useful feedback from the person they are treating than would be the case if they were practising on a non-Reiki-attuned volunteer.

Reiki practice days are also suitable for people who learned Reiki some time ago and now want to get back into treating other people, and would like a bit of advice or support before unleashing themselves again on friends and family, and the general public!

What do people get out of such a day?

Two things: confidence and reassurance.

You create a safe place where people are all there to help and support each other, and you provide helpful and supportive comments, suggesting things, confirming that students are doing things well and can trust any impressions that they may be having about where to spend longer during a treatment, say, or in terms of where they feel they need to rest their hands.

You can encourage them when they are feeling the energy field or scanning, and reassure them that they don't need to worry about 'getting things wrong'.

Students can have their questions and nagging doubts dealt with: things may have occurred to them since their course that they were wondering about but they didn't want to bother their teacher about that, and you can deal with those things face-to-face.

Or things may happen during their supervised treatments that prompt them to ask questions that they had forgotten they wanted to ask about.

Of course, no-one has answers to every question about Reiki, and sometimes the answer might be "no-one knows" or "nobody knows and it doesn't matter anyway"; it can be useful for people to hear that.

What you will need

You will need a venue, of course, big enough to accommodate one treatment table for every 2-3 participants.

You'll need something that you can play some background music on, and it is nice to have refreshments on hand.

Partly this can be a social occasion where students talk to and support each other, and you can facilitate this.

Here's a possible format

Energy exercises:

Start by talking everyone through Hatsurei ho (or Kenyoku followed by Joshin Kokkyu ho), or you can play the "Reiki Meditations" audio CD or MP3 track, so you can join in too!

Empowerments:

While everyone is sitting quietly, you can go round giving everyone simple Reiju empowerments.

Sharing experiences:

Encourage participants to talk about their experiences of working on other people. What amazed them, what puzzled or concerned them, what doubts or questions do they have about what they have experienced thus far when using Reiki on themselves and other people?

Treat others under supervision:

Students then treat each other in pairs or groups of three.

As a group you can talk them through the beginning of a treatment: the ACBMF sequence, you can suggest the feeling of the energy field and scanning, as you would on a First Degree course, but in an abbreviated way (you're not here to teach people things for the first time: you're here to remind and encourage them!) and then you can let them carry on with the treatment as they wish.

You are on hand all the time, you can move from table to table, occasionally suggesting things; by being available and close by, students are likely to call you over to ask you something about what they are doing or experiencing.

Feedback:

Once all the treatments have finished, you can all get together as a group and ask people for feedback about what they found interesting or useful, what they noticed or experienced (giving the treatment or being the recipient) and any 'aha' moments that they had and want to share.

You can pick up on different comments and use them as brief 'teaching points', but this is not a big teaching session: just make a few useful and positive points to keep people focused on the main issues and principles. You don't want to disappear down an obscure side-alley!

Co-ordinating treatments given by two people

If your students end in a group of three when treating each other, with one person lying on the treatment table and the others treating them, they may need some guidance as to how to work this.

This is what can happen:

Both 'treaters' can spend a little while feeling the recipient's energy field and doing a bit of scanning.

Then one sits down at the head of the table while the other stands by the recipient's torso, as you can see in the illustration below.

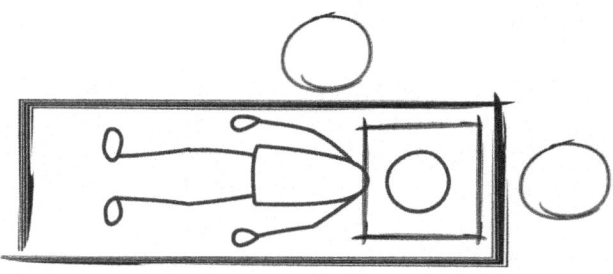

The person sitting at the head of the table can start with the head/shoulders for a while, to get the energy flowing and to make the recipient all relaxed and open to the energy.

Then they move on to treat the (1) crown, (2) temples, (3) back of head, (4) front of face, and (5) throat positions.

At the same time, the person standing by the table can start with the heart/solar plexus for a while, for a longer period than they will spend on the subsequent hand positions.

Then they move on to treat the (1) abdomen, (2) hips, (3) thighs, (4) knees, and (5) ankles positions.

As the treatment finishes, the standing person smooths down the energy field and both treaters 'disconnect'.

Giving advice to students

Students' questions and doubts will probably revolve around these sorts of issues:

1. Hand positions
2. Feeling the energy field
3. Scanning
4. Interpreting different sensations
5. Wondering whether their intuition is working

You are there to provide reassurance that they do not need to follow the instructions to the letter for fear of the treatment or their Reiki 'not working' in some way: that the energy is flexible and accommodates many different approaches and ways of working.

You will spend your time reassuring them that they can trust what they are feeling in their hands (whether that means a particularly strong or interesting sensation... or a lack of any sensation in a particular area).

And you will encourage them to accept and trust what they are noticing intuitively: whether they feel strangely drawn to work on a particular area, or to stay for longer in a particular area, or whether they feel that their hands are drifting to a particular place.

You can help them by doing some quick scanning yourself, or feeling the energy field, to confirm that you are picking up a similar thing.

Explain that people's sensations can differ, and while they may feel heat or buzzing, you have a different but broadly equivalent sensation.

And you can quickly see where your hands want to drift to, to confirm that you agree with what is coming to them intuitively, or to confirm that there's not much of an intuitive pull anywhere for this particular recipient.

Sometimes it is important or useful to be able to say to someone "no, there's nothing interesting to notice here", so the message they receive is "you're not missing something here because there's nothing to notice... so you were right!"

How Reiki Evolution can help with your courses

Did you know that people all over the world are using Reiki Evolution course manuals and audio CDs on their Reiki courses? And not just people who have trained with Reiki Evolution: people from all Reiki lineages and styles.

The reason for that is that I seem to have put together some resources that aren't available anywhere else (from what I have seen):

Reiki manuals

I have created professionally printed and bound course manuals that are detailed, comprehensive and easy to read, containing careful descriptions, images and summaries that make it easy for students to get to grips with all the main practices of Reiki healing. I have manuals for you to use as follows (all A4 size):

- Reiki First Degree (Shoden) – 170 pages
- Reiki Second Degree (Okuden) – 110 pages
- Reiki Master Teacher (Shinpiden) – 230 pages

Read what Sherry Coffman, a Reiki Master Teacher from Texas, USA, thinks about Reiki Evolution course manuals:

"When I first started my journey with Reiki, I was not provided with a manual of any kind. I was given a resource list and a folder with some handouts. My original Reiki Master Teacher was unable to complete the Master level training with me due to personal illness and so I had to move on to another Master Teacher.

It turned out to be the best thing that could have happened for me because the new Master was using Taggart King's manuals. So, I was introduced to the materials with Shinpiden. When I decided to begin conducting my own trainings, I reviewed First Degree with my new Master. That's when I saw the Shoden manual for the first time. At that point I was hooked and now I provide the appropriate level manual for my students as part of their training.

"Using Taggart's manuals fits my personality as a teacher. They are direct, complete and give full explanations with visuals for anything that a blooming practitioner could need. I especially love his sense of humor and the way he brings a reality to every day Reiki while still holding a space of total respect for the wisdom and mystery of Reiki.

"He speaks with the voice of authority, but encourages students to be guided by personal intuition. I especially

appreciate his commitment to researching and sharing the original Japanese ways, making it clear where and how Western Reiki traditions have entered the scene.

"Using his materials gives me confidence as a teacher knowing my students have a quality manual to which they can refer in the days following their training."

Reiki audio CDs

You will have seen from the various articles that I have written that I believe it is important to provide students with course materials that meet their different learning styles, and how important it is to provide comprehensive training materials that students can revisit after their training day.

Reiki audio CDs help with this a great deal because they can listen to a potted version of a Reiki course – hearing the main points of what they would hear on a live training day – and also be guided through the main energy exercises and meditations and self-treatments that we teach.

So I have audio CDs for you that either provide commentary (like listening to a live course) or guided meditations:

- Reiki First Degree commentary
- Reiki Second Degree commentary

- "Reiki Meditations" (suitable for First and Second Degree and consists of: Hatsurei ho, Self-treatment meditation, Symbol meditation and Distant healing session)
- "Talking you through a Reiki treatment" – does what it says on the tin! – talks you through a full, hour-long Reiki treatment.
- Reiki Master Teacher commentary
- Reiki Master Teacher guided instructions (talks you through a Reiki attunement, a Japanese Reiju empowerment, a session where you open to intuition (the Japanese 'Reiji ho' method) and a special 'Frequency scale' meditation that Taggart devised

Reiki Certificate templates

I know that one of the things that can be quite challenging to begin with, when you start running your own Reiki courses, is to get together decent-looking Reiki certificates.

To help people with this I enlisted the help of a Japanese Calligraphy Master, who has brushed for me a traditional Japanese certificate, using Japanese calligraphy, that can be used for any Reiki course or training.

I have put together Reiki certificate templates that you can download or order on DVD-rom. They come in different formats and with all the special kanji that you would need to create gorgeous Japanese-style certificates for your students.

See what some Reiki Masters thought of the Reiki certificate templates:

"I have now used the CD Rom that you supplied to me for making Reiki Certificates. I have used it on two occasions and found it easy to use and the end result is good and looks very professional. I liked the fact that I could choose different wordings re attunements, empowerments, initiations. Thank you for making this available: without it I would, no doubt, be floundering around wondering how to do it!"

Sally Beautista, London

"I used the Reiki Certificates CD-ROM for a Reiki 1 course last weekend, which I ran on a one/one for a lady who wanted to learn Reiki to use on her farm animals. Not being 'into' computers apart from emails etc. I was very pleased with the certificate I produced with your CD."

Geraldine Shuttleworth, Staffordshire

"The Certificates CD I received was extremely good value for money. I did make some amendments to personalise my certificates as you suggested. Another fantastic resource with step by step instructions for the technophobes amongst us (I am referring to myself of

course!). Anyone that has any of your other CD's will know how the energy flows when they are played and this resource CD is no different. It set my creative side alight! I was instinctively drawn to the CD and you did not disappoint."

Caron Sanders-Crook, London

I am very pleased with the CD-ROM it has been very useful to have a template, especially a choice of templates to work with. I am not that computer literate so it was nice to be able to produce something that looks so professional."

Rachel Robinson, West Midlands

106

Discounts for ordering resources in 'multipacks'

I have put together packs of 4 Reiki manuals or CDs that you can order at reduced prices.

I have priced the packs so that you receive a discount of 33% compared with retail price (First Degree manual) and a discount of 50% for the audio CDs.

When you order the Reiki manuals, I arrange for them to be specially printed for you and they go in the post to you in a couple of days, whether that's in the UK, USA, Canada, Australia, or anywhere else in the world.

I post you your audio CDs the next working day, and they are mainly ordered by UK Reiki teachers.

Here is the web page where you can order discounted packs of books and manuals:

http://www.reiki-evolution.co.uk/buying-in-bulk/

Below you can read some comments from other Reiki Masters who are using Reiki Evolution course materials:

"I have used Reiki Evolution course materials for some time. It is a pleasure to use them as they are clear and comprehensive, easy to follow with clear diagrams and instructions.

"All materials are produced to a high specification – creating an image of professionalism. The manuals are a good reference for students to browse through, enabling them to reflect and digest all that has been given and shown to them.

"The CDs too, assist with all aspects covered including meditations. For those students with dyslexia the CDs have proved very popular."

Oonagh Van Hemuss, Reiki Master Teacher

"I have been using Reiki Evolution resources ever since I started running my own courses and teaching Reiki. This is mainly because I don't believe in re-inventing wheels! There is such depth of information in the manuals, even if I wanted to, I could not produce anything better myself.

"From a personal point of view, I return to the manuals time and time again to refresh my knowledge and check what I may have overlooked. I really like the fact that within the manuals there are options and little is set in stone. I can choose for myself which approaches to take both when self treating and when giving a Reiki treatment so I can choose the techniques which work best for me. Re-visiting the manuals gives me the opportunity to find techniques I've left aside and try them when I'm ready to. This is very much the approach I suggest to all my Reiki students.

"There is always positive feedback from people on my Reiki courses about both the manuals and the CDs. As a teacher of Reiki, it is great having such excellent resources readily available to distribute.

"People who book on my courses have often trained to level 1 or 2 with another Reiki lineage so I always ask to see any manuals or support materials they have been given. This allows me to see the similarities across the courses and where I might wish to include additional elements on the course.

Whilst there are some good support materials out there, to date, no other manual has come close to the depth of the manuals provided by Reiki Evolution. In fact, in many cases there have been no support materials or 'manuals' that consist of around 10 pages of large font containing only a small amount of information. With the Reiki Evolution manual there is no need to flounder after the course and struggle to remember everything as it can be referred to time and time again.

"In my experience, very few other lineages distribute CDs as part of their courses. Reiki Evolution CDs are a great aid to learning and back up information in each manual. They can be played in the background or in the car until all of the information is absorbed, or used in a more structured way as the pre-course study course is followed. The CDs also serve as a good refresher after the course.

"The meditation CDs are excellent and help to quickly get the listener relaxed and reach a meditative state…backed up by endless comments from my Reiki students about how much they love Taggart's voice. Occasionally I get approached by previous students who have not given Reiki much attention for a while – the meditation CD can help people to find their way back to Reiki.

"Many people, years after they have completed their Reiki courses tell me they still use the meditation CD regularly…it's easy, it works so why not?

Rhonda Bailey, Reiki Master Teacher

A WORD ABOUT REIKI INITIATIONS AND WHAT THEY ARE

Introduction

No matter what Reiki lineage you trained in, you will have received some sort of an initiation – probably more than one – on each Reiki course you attended. The ritual that you went through might have been quite brief or it may have been quite elaborate and detailed, it may have been referred to as an 'attunement' or it could have been called an 'empowerment'.

Before you experienced this 'mystical hand-waiving' you couldn't do Reiki... and afterwards you could.

For many people the initiation to Reiki is like going through a very special and profound experience and then flipping on a switch, a switch that leads within minutes to being able to feel sensations in your hands that you weren't aware of before or, if you were aware of them, were not noticeable with such intensity. People tell you that your hands feel burning hot when you get them near to someone, yet they can at the same time be cool to the touch.

What is going on here?

We are said to have been 'attuned' to something.

But what?...

Do we connect at all?

It all starts with a connection, doesn't it? We "attune" to the energy, connecting them or hooking them up to a source of energy that they did not have access to before... or do we?

Are we connecting people to something external to them?

One of the important principles of the original system was the concept of 'oneness' and in fact one of the goals of the original system was to experience this state, by working with meditations and/or kotodama at Second Degree.

The idea here is that what we experience as reality is said to be 'illusion' : the notion that we are individuals, separate and distinct from other people, is an illusion, and ultimate reality is oneness.

There is no me, there is no you. In fact one way that you could explain distant healing is by saying that there is no problem in 'sending' the energy to another person because there is no other person and there is no you!

And in that light, how could there be something external to us that we 'connect' to, how could there be something that we were not 'at one' with: we already have the connection.

So what does the attunement do?

Well we could see the ritual as a way of directing the student's attention in a particular way, helping them to recognise or notice something that has always been there.

I like to explain this in these terms:

Imagine that you are visiting a friend and you walk into their lounge. They say to you, "can you hear that high-pitched noise?". You can't hear anything, well not to begin with, anyway.

Then you listen, you really listen, you focus your attention in a new way, in a different way from how you were paying attention when you first walked into the room... and suddenly you can hear the sound because you have 'tuned in' to it.

You have been 'attuned' to something that had already been there, and you were only attuned to that sound through the intervention of your friend, who asked you the right question.

And to take this metaphor a little further, does it matter exactly what wording your friend uses to direct your attention to the sound that you couldn't initially hear?

No, of course not, there are many ways of asking someone to pay attention to a 'mystery' sound.

Your friend needed to be there in some way to facilitate the process, but the detail of what they said isn't so important.

Their intention in directing your attention in a particular way is what's significant.

And in fact they didn't even need to have been in the room: they could have called you on the telephone and asked the question, or they could have left you a note to read.

The end result would have been the same: the intervention of a third party, in some way, helping you to 'tune in' to something that had already existed and which you had the potential to experience, but didn't until your friend helped to point you in the right direction in terms of your awareness.

Where are attunements from?

It seems fairly clear that Usui Sensei did not attune anyone to anything: he did not use attunements. He empowered people using intent. Attunements only came into being after Usui's death when the Imperial Officers got together and created a ritual that gave them the same sort of experiences that they had noticed when being empowered by Usui.

They had only trained with Usui for a relatively short space of time and would not have reached the level where they would have been taught how to empower others, so they put together their own ritual.

And what was this ritual, exactly? Well, it's difficult to say. There is information about a ritual that Tatsumi was taught by Dr Hayashi, but there is some disagreement about exactly what the ritual was for.

Dr Hayashi will have taught attunements to Mrs Takata, and one assumes that she passed these on in an unmodified form to the teachers that she initiated but, as I understand it, even within "The Reiki Alliance" – an organisation greatly wedded to the Office of Grandmaster – the attunement rituals have been altered and modified in different lineages.

There is a notion that you have to have four attunements for First Degree for it to be 'kosher', though in some lineages they might carry out three, or two, or even one.

Various principles from different energetic systems have been slotted into Reiki over the years, and symbols from non-Reiki sources, too. So, for example, the attunements that Reiki Evolution use, which are slightly mutated 'William Rand' attunements, include the 'Tibetan' Master Symbol, and also the use of the HuiYin, the Fire Dragon and the Violet breath.

We are taught three different First Degree attunements, but we do the third one twice to make that magic number four!

Not all Reiki teachers have the 'Tibetan' Master symbol, not all use the violet breath, not all connect the HuiYin, not all use the magic 'four' attunements approach, and the empowerments used by Usui's surviving students did not involve using any of these things.

So I suggest that if we're going to carry out attunements then we use the method that we were taught, and make sure that we are doing it 'correctly', while also remembering that the individual details of a particular attunement style are not so important.

You are there as a facilitator, someone who helps the student to recognise something that is already there within them, and this can be achieved in different ways.

Distant connections

There is controversy about the use of distant attunements and, currently, none of the Reiki associations will accept students that have received distant attunements, only 'in person' ones.

None of the societies have specified what is the maximum safe distance that a teacher has to be from the student in order for an attunement to qualify.

This aversion to distant attunements involves amazing mental gymnastics: on the one hand such people believe that Reiki can be sent from one side of the planet to another, to the future, to the past, just by thinking about it (or by using a symbol and thinking about it), passing through the planet... and yet when it comes to 'connection' rituals the teacher has to stand right in front of the student otherwise it won't work.

Of course a lot of online Reiki courses are rubbish, but that can also be said of many 'in person' Reiki courses, where students emerge with no clear idea of what Reiki is, nor how to use it for their own benefit or to treat others..

Attunements or empowerments?

There are further controversies, of course. As I understand it, the UKRF (UK Reiki Federation) will not allow you to upgrade your membership to 'Practitioner' status unless you have received attunements on your Second Degree course because of its apparent belief that empowerments do not attune you to Reiki.

This means, of course – and this is a ridiculous situation for Reiki to have gotten into - that no-one taught by Mikao Usui would qualify for a 'Practitioner' upgrade.

Let's just say that again: none of the people taught by the founder of Reiki would be good enough to receive 'practitioner' status with the UKRF!

You couldn't make it up.

So they seem to be framing Reiki as being something that derives from the Imperial Officers, not from Mikao Usui.

You can't get in unless you've had an attunement, and of course these were only available after Usui's death.

If you trained with Reiki Evolution as a Master Teacher, you probably won't be using attunements so often since you'll most likely choose to use Reiju empowerments instead.

I recommend that you use attunements on any RMT courses that you run so that, as far as the 'blinkered and dogmatic' Reiki community is concerned, your RMT students have been 'properly' connected, and if you wanted to make sure that your Second Degree courses meet the UKRF dogma test then you'd use attunements for Second Degree courses too.

But I don't recommend that: not everyone who learns Reiki wants to become a practitioner and join the UKRF, so once in a blue moon you might be contacted by a student about this issue; just arrange for them to receive an attunement from you and give them a piece of paper that certifies that.

Just to be clear: both attunements and empowerments 'connect' you to Reiki, permanently.

The Reiki Evolution attunement method

If you attended a Reiki Evolution RMT (Reiki Master Teacher) course you were taught how to carry out a Second Degree attunement because starting with these attunements first is about the most logical way to do it: getting the Reiki 2 attunements set in your head first, and then seeing how these differ from Master attunements and First Degree attunements.

You have a range of materials that you can use to get to grips with the process: written descriptions, summaries, drawings, little cards that you shuffle and put in order, photographs, a video sequence and an audio track that talks you through the process.

By way of comparison, most people who learn attunements on a Master course receive a demo on their live course and have written instructions of variable quality, so if you trained with Reiki Evolution you have absolutely everything that you need to get to grips with the process.

Use whichever combination of materials suits your learning style.

In the Reiki Evolution system, Master attunements don't differ greatly from Second Degree attunements. It's the First Degree attunements that differ the most, and you probably won't be using these unless you feel particularly drawn to using attunements; if you really like attunements then please go ahead and use them.

Attunements are certainly a 'High Church' ritual, but some people are attracted to a 'big event', and that's fine: we don't all have to be the same!

To begin with, when learning how to carry out attunements, you will of necessity be focused on the individual stages, making sure that you remember everything and carry things out in the right sequence.

You can practise on an empty chair, on a large teddy bear, or on a long-suffering Reiki friend.

With practice the sequences will become more fluid and seamless, you'll think less about what you're doing, and things will start to flow nicely.

With practice you can 'get out of the way' and maintain a nice, empty, merged state, more an observer of the ritual than a participant in it.

That's the sort of state that you're looking to achieve.

The individual stages of attunements

We know that attunement rituals have mutated and altered as they have been passed on from teacher to teacher, and some of the changes will simply reflect that teacher's particular style of working, where they have expressed their intention – or their understanding of what is going on when you 'attune' someone – in terms of a particular hand or arm movement, a particular affirmation or visualization.

The outer ritual expresses an inner intention, and an intention can be expressed in different ways by different people.

Of course, people have come to different conclusions about what they are doing and why, based on their belief systems and other practices that they are involved with, so teachers will have conflicting beliefs about what is a necessary part of an attunement, what needs to be carried out for an attunement to be effective.

There are many attunement styles, reflecting differing belief systems, and these conflicting attunements work.

They work because they are all expressions of an intention, which underpins what you are doing when you 'attune'.

WHY REIKI EVOLUTION COURSES ARE THE WAY THEY ARE

Introduction

It is clear that what Mikao Usui was teaching to the majority of his students was quite different from the system that he passed on to the Imperial Officers, who approached Usui Sensei to be taught a hands-on healing system that could be used in the Imperial Navy.

What Usui had been teaching to most of his students was a self-healing and spiritual development system that didn't focus very much on working on other people: it was a "system to achieve personal perfection".

Dr Hayashi modified what he had been taught and, correctly, renamed what he was teaching as Hayashi Reiki (Hayashi Reiki Kenyukai). He passed on his system to Mrs Takata and she initiated Masters in the 1970s, passing on to them what she thought appropriate.

Since then, Reiki has travelled through the New Age movement and assimilated such things as chakra work, spirit guides, crystals, Angels, and influences from other healing systems, for example spiritual healing, and the beliefs that are attached to these other ways of working with energy.

Reiki has changed, altered, mutated in different lineages and, ironically, while most people say that they practice

"Traditional Usui" Reiki, in fact what they are doing is non-traditional and fairly non-Usui too!

So what I am going to talk about in this section is (1) What Mikao Usui seems to have taught and (2) How we echo the original system that Usui was teaching on Reiki Evolution courses, so far as that's possible in the Western 'weekend course' format.

We don't know exactly what Usui taught, not everything he taught is really suitable for a Western audience, and some of the ways that the original system was taught doesn't really fit very well with the way that Reiki is taught in the West.

We're not going to set up a dojo, we're not going to be having students studying Buddhist sutras or chanting Japanese poetry, and some of the energy exercises that the original students carried out early on in their Reiki training would be counterproductive to introduce at such an early stage, in my opinion. So what I have done is to mould the original approaches and practices into a format that seems to work.

Below we will take a look at what Usui taught to most of his students, compare that in detail with what's taught on many Western-style Reiki courses (a rough approximation anyway, since there are lots of different Western Reiki variations) and then we'll move on to see how I decided to present the original practices in a 'Western' training format.

What Mikao Usui taught

The information that we have about the original system comes from Chris Marsh, via a group of Usui's surviving students who were in contact with him. Arjava Petter has uncovered a few of the component parts, and some of the basic practices of the Gakkai - as passed on by Hiroshi Doi - echo Reiki in its original form. But Gakkai Reiki is not original Usui Reiki, whether it has come to us via Petter or Doi.

The thing that strikes me most about original Usui Reiki is the fact that it is so simple, so elegant, powerful and uncluttered. The system is not bogged down in endless mechanical techniques and complex rituals.

The prime focus of Mikao Usui's Reiki is the personal benefits that will come through committing oneself to working with the system, both in terms of self-healing and spiritual development. Reiki was a path to enlightenment.

Healing others was a minor aspect of the system, not emphasised, not focused upon; it was simply something that you could do if you followed Usui's system.

Original Usui Reiki involves committing yourself to carrying out daily energy exercises, treating yourself (a range of approaches were available) and receiving spiritual empowerments on a regular basis.

You learned to work with meditations or ancient Shinto mantras that represent different aspects of the energy, and you did this to further your self-healing and spiritual development; these mantras could also be used when treating others.

There were very few treatment techniques and the focus was very much on intuition; symbols did not enter into the process for the vast majority of Usui Sensei's students and were only introduced for the Imperial Officers in about 1923; Usui had been teaching his system since at least 1915.

Original Usui Reiki gives all of us the chance to maximise our Reiki potential. We can practice exercises that make us a strong clear channel for Reiki; we can learn to 'become' two important energies, and to experience 'oneness'.

And when we treat others, we can learn to open to intuition so that the energy moves our hands to just the right places to treat in each person we work on.

Simple. Elegant. Powerful.

Let's get three revelations out of the way to begin with:

1.   Usui's system wasn't called Reiki
2.   Usui's system wasn't about treating people
3.   Usui's system didn't use symbols

Usui's System wasn't Called Reiki

The first revelation about original Usui Reiki is that it was not called 'Reiki', in fact Usui's system had no name. Usui seems to have referred to the system as either 'My system' or 'Method to Achieve Personal Perfection'.

His students seem to have referred to the system as 'Usui Teate' or 'Usui Do'.

The word Reiki appears in the Reiki precepts, but the word 'Reiki' there seems to mean 'a system that has been arrived at through a moment of enlightenment', or 'a gift of satori'.

The name 'Reiki' came later, and may have been used first when the naval officers, his less-experienced students, set up the Usui Reiki Ryoho Gakkai after Usui's death.

The teachings that are coming from Usui's surviving students were referred to as 'Usui Teate' by Chris Marsh and his associate Andrew Bowling, and you may come across this phrase.

129

The word 'teate' should be pronounced 'tee-ah-tay' with emphasis on the first and last syllables. Teate means 'hand healing' or 'hand application', and there is a hundreds of years old tradition of Japanese hand healing techniques that work on he recipient's chi, perhaps similar to QiGong healing techniques.

Usui's System wasn't about Treating People

The next revelation is that the purpose of Usui's method was to achieve satori, to find one's spiritual path, to heal oneself. Usui's system was not really about treating others.

Treating others was not emphasised; it was not focused upon; it was a side issue.

Usui's system was a spiritual system and his teachings in terms of treating others amounted to "you can do this". Some students were taught some standard hand positions to use when treating the head, and some weren't. The approach was basically intuitive, and any suggested hand-positions were a stopgap.

With time the students would move on to treat intuitively, or would carry out 'intention' healings, where they would connect to the recipient and the healing would take place during whatever period was appropriate.

Once the initial connection was made, the healing could take place no matter what the 'healer' then went on to do: there was no need to concentrate on the recipient.

The initial connection/intention was the thing that led to the healing taking place.

Usui's System didn't use Symbols

As far as the vast majority of Usui Sensei's students are concerned, the system did not involve the use of symbols: they were never taught to use symbols and they were not attuned to symbols.

What we refer to as the Reiki symbols were introduced by Usui Sensei and his senior student Eguchi as a quick way of depicting the energies, introduced for the benefit of the Imperial officers who approached Usui in order to learn a hands-on healing system that they could use within the Japanese military.

Even then, Usui Sensei did not attune the Imperial Officers to the symbols: they were simply a visual focus that was used to elicit/invoke a particular energy.

The other students had used either meditations or chanted Shinto mantras to learn to experience or become a particular energy or a state.

The Origins of Usui's System

The system was rooted in Tendai Buddhism, Shintoism and Shugendo (mountain asceticism). Tendai Buddhism (a form of mystical Buddhism) provided spiritual teachings and spiritual empowerments, Shintoism contributed methods of controlling and working with the energies, and Shugendo provided the precepts on which Usui based his own.

Usui had a strong background in both kiko (energy cultivation) and a martial art with a strong Zen flavour (Yagyu Shinkage Ryu), and he also took Soto Zen training for a while, and these studies may have contributed in some way to the system that he developed, and certainly contributed to his own spiritual development.

The system was based on living and practising the Reiki principles; that was the hub of the whole thing.

The vast majority of Usui's students started out as his clients, people who came to him because they wanted something treated.

He would routinely give people empowerments (connect them to Reiki) so that they could treat themselves in between appointments with him, and if they wanted to take things further then they could start formal training.

The training was rather like martial arts training: you had an open-ended commitment to study with Usui, not a fixed-length training course, the teachings were geared towards the student's individual needs, and it was only when the student had developed sufficiently that they were invited to move on to higher levels.

It is important to emphasise that to refer to what Usui Sensei was passing on as 'a system' suggests that there were fixed teachings that were passed on in the same way to all his students.

This was not the case: he modified his teachings according to the background and needs of his students, as individuals, so some students were given one set of approaches and worked in one particular way, while others were provided with other approaches.

Having said that, here you can read about Usui Sensei's general approaches at each training 'level'...

Usui's First Degree (Shoden)

First Degree (Shoden) was very simple, and it seems that Usui taught hundreds of people at this level.

Shoden was all about opening to the energy through receiving empowerments, it was about cleansing and self-healing.

1. Students would receive Reiju empowerments from Usui Sensei again and again. In fact this continued through all levels.

2. The students would carry out simple energy exercises each day. The exercises taught at first-degree level were Kenyoku and Joshin Kokkyu Ho, which are taught in the Usui Reiki Ryoho Gakkai as part of a longer sequence of exercises called 'Hatsurei ho'.

3. The student would practise self-healing; there were different approaches available, including self-healing meditations.

4. Students would chant and live Usui Sensei's precepts.

5. Students would study some specially selected 'Waka' poems, chosen by Usui

because they contained various sacred sounds (kotodama).

6. Students would be introduced to the concept of mindfulness.

In anticipation of moving on to Second Degree level, students would have to focus on developing their awareness of their hara; only when they had successfully defined their hara would they move on to the next level. We will talk about this more later.

Students would not treat others at first-degree.

A Little about the Precepts

Everyone who has learned Reiki will have seen the precepts, and they are available in a variety of different forms.

There is actually some difference between the precepts that Mikao Usui was teaching and the precepts that are quoted commonly in the West, so perhaps we should start by reading the text of Usui Sensei's version:

> The secret of inviting happiness through many blessings*
> The spiritual medicine for all illness
>
> For today only: Do not anger; Do not worry

Be humble
Be honest in your work**

Be compassionate to yourself and others

Do gassho every morning and evening
Keep in your mind and recite

The phrase "many blessings" is likely to refer to Reiju empowerments (the 'attunement' method used by Mikao Usui and the surviving students), so it really means "The secret of inviting happiness through receiving many Reiju empowerments", and of course students who trained with Usui Sensei would receive empowerments again and again throughout their training at all levels.

The phrase "be honest in your work" really means "be honest in your dealings with people".

You will note that there is no precept that exhorts us to "honour our parents, elders and teachers".

This seems to have been added to the list, perhaps by Mrs Takata, to make the "list of rules to live by" more acceptable to her American audience.

There has been some speculation about where Mikao Usui's precepts come from. It has been claimed that they originate in a book that was published in Usui's time, and it has been claimed that they are based on the edicts of Mutsuhito, the Meiji Emperor.

Certainly it seems that many Tendai and Zen Buddhist teachers were passing on similar principles in Usui Sensei's time.

But we now know that Usui's precepts were his wording of an earlier set of precepts that have been traced back to the early 9th Century, precepts which were used in a Tendai sect of Shugendo with which Usui Sensei was in contact.

These earlier precepts were the basic daily practice and rule in Shugendo.

The precepts were the baseline, the foundation of Usui Sensei's teachings, and it was thought that individual could achieve as much spiritual development by following the precepts as could be achieved by carrying out all the energy exercises.

The principles really are the 'hub' of the whole system.

Usui's Second Degree (Okuden)

Second Degree (Okuden) was split into two levels (Zenki and Kouki). Perhaps 70 students reached Zenki, with 30 of these reaching Kouki level.

Second-degree was all about strengthening your ability as a channel, becoming familiar with some specific energies and a particular state of mind, and receiving spiritual teachings.

You became a stronger channel for Reiki by receiving Reiju empowerments on a regular basis, and by practising energy exercises. Reiju continually reinforced your connection to the source and allowed you to grow spiritually.

You would work on that renewed connection by doing daily energy exercises which took a different form from those carried out at first-degree.

The Spiritual teachings introduced at Second Degree level involved studying Buddhist sutras, specifically the Lotus sutra, the Heart sutra and the Diamond sutra. The Lotus sutra is the foundation document of Tendai Buddhism.

Though one source of 'original' information claims that Usui became a Shingon Buddhist, his surviving students insist that he was 'Tendai to the end'. The fact that he was Tendai did not stop him from drawing from other spiritual traditions in Japan though.

Mindfulness would be emphasised more at this level.

Zenki

In the first of the two second-degree levels (Zenki) you would practise 'becoming' the energies that in the West we use ChoKuRei and SeiHeKi to represent: these energies are seen as earth Ki and heavenly Ki by the surviving students.

You would do this by practising various meditations over many months, or by meditating on sacred sounds, or maybe a bit of both approaches. You learned to 'become' these energies over an extended period of time in order to move along your path to enlightenment, and to promote self-healing.

This process was not rushed, since you had to learn to 'become' the energies fully, one energy at a time.

Students would have worked with each aspect of the energy for maybe 6-9 months before moving on, so it was a slow process.

The sacred sounds that you used to further your self-healing and spiritual development could also be used to treat others, and students might do some treatments at this level, though it was a bit of a sideline to the main thrust of the system.

Treatments might be based on a few simple hand positions that were used on the head, though this was not taught to all students, and the focus was very much on intuition in terms of hand-placement and in terms of what energy – if any – you emphasised during the treatment.

The sacred sounds, called 'Kotodama' (or 'Jumon' if referred to from a Buddhist perspective), come from Shintoism, the indigenous religion of Japan.

This is really ancient stuff. This takes us back to the mists of ancient Japanese history, to a time when the sound of the human voice was said to be able to stop armies, to kill, to heal and to control the weather.

There were three kotodama, or jumon, taught at second degree, representing the three energies that in the West we use the symbols to represent.

The two energies that were introduced at Okuden Zenki and had to be fully integrated before you moved on to Okuden Kouki.

Kouki

At the second of the two second-degree levels (Kouki) you would be introduced to the concept of oneness, one of the goals of the system, and learn through meditations, and/or the use of a Kotodama, to fully experience oneness.

Distance healing is an expression of oneness, and students would have realised that they could do this easily.

In fact treating others is an expression of oneness too!

Treatment Techniques

All the other 'Usui' techniques that are practised by the Usui Reiki Ryoho Gakkai (the Japanese association that carries Usui's name) and have been passed to us through Arjava Petter and Hiroshi Doi are in fact not original 'Usui Teate' techniques, but seem to be mostly Japanese QiGong techniques contained in a QiGong manual that was published in 1927 by the Japanese Navy and issued to all Imperial Officers.

No doubt Usui knew of these techniques, because he had practised kiko, but they were not part of his system.

Meditations

The interesting thing about the meditations that Usui taught to his students is that it was only when the students had become completely familiar with the energies that they were given a 'trigger' to connect to what they already had strongly within them.

In the West we use a symbol to connect to an energy that is unfamiliar to us; in Usui's system you became familiar with an energy and then were given a way of triggering it.

No symbols entered into Usui's system for most of his students, and thus the empowerments (connection rituals) do not use symbols either; why would they, since Usui's system was up and running long before he introduced symbols for the benefit of Dr Hayashi and the other naval officers in 1923.

Usui seems to have taught his system as early as 1915, maybe even earlier.

Usui's Master levels (Shinpiden and Shihan)

The Master levels (Shinpiden and Shihan) involved receiving further spiritual teachings, receiving Reiju and other 'higher' empowerments, and learning how to empower yourself.

You were introduced to a further kotodama, and you practised a whole series of meditations, or energy exercises, that built on each other and were designed to move you further along your spiritual path and closer and closer to your own satori.

Satori is not the same as the Sanskrit 'nirvana' or spiritual bliss where you experience unity with the divine; it is not a one-time once-and-for-all experience.

Satori is a moment of recognition, when you have a flash of insight that changes something in a fundamental way. It would come through a long period of meditation; it is something that you have to work at, by getting rid of your 'baggage'.

Eventually, near the end of your Master training, you learned how to perform Reiju and other 'higher' empowerments. This may have been described as 'Shihan' level rather than 'Shinpiden' (mystery teachings).

The system was open-ended though: you never completed it; it was a lifetime journey. It was about defining and finding your place cosmically.

It took as long as it took, through continued practice.

Comparing Western and Original Reiki

What I want to do now is to compare the way that Reiki is usually taught on standard 'Western' Hayashi/Takata Reiki courses with what we know of Mikao Usui's original system.

I have put the information into some tables for easy reference and then summarised the main differences below each table.

Differences

So the main differences (see below) between standard Western Reiki and the original system at First Degree are that while Western Reiki is focuses on treating yourself to an extent and treating others to a greater extent, the original system omits the treatment of others and focuses on self-development/spiritual-development using a variety of energy approaches, the practice of mindfulness, the study of Waka poetry and through living the precepts.

First Degree

Western Reiki	Original system
Receive attunements (usually 4)	Receive empowerments repeatedly. Usui used intention
	Practise mindfulness
A version of the precepts taught, usually including 'honour your parents, teachers & elders'	Chant and live Usui's precepts
History of Reiki	
	Kenyoku/Joshin Kokkyu ho
Hands-on self-treatment method	Practise self-healing, different approaches, for example the USTM* or 'meditate with the intention to heal'
	Study special waka poetry, chosen by Usui because of kotodama contained within it; we don't know what these were
Treat other people	

*USTM = "Usui Self-Treatment Meditation" where you imagine that you are treating yourself by focusing the energy on different areas of your head.

Second Degree

Western Reiki	Original system
Receive attunement(s)	Receive empowerments repeatedly. Usui used intention.
	Mindfulness emphasised more
	Studying Lotus, Heart and Diamond sutras
Learn CKR symbol and various symbol sandwiches	Become earth ki for 6-9 months at 'Zenki' level: Buddhist-style meditations or kotodama chanting. No symbols taught.
Learn SHK symbol and various symbol sandwiches	Become earth ki for 6-9 months at 'Zenki' level: Buddhist-style meditations or kotodama chanting. No symbols taught.
Learn HSZSN symbol	Some students moved on to 'Kouki' level to experience oneness Meditation ('breath of being') or kotodama chanting used. No symbols
Distant healing practised	
Using symbols when treating others	Maybe some treatment of others; maybe a few hand positions, mostly intuition. No symbols

147

There were two sub-levels in the original system. 70 people achieved the first level (Zenki), and 30 reached the second level (Kouki), where you got to grips with oneness.

Students with a Buddhist background used meditations to get to grips with earth ki, heavenly ki and oneness, and then they were given the kotodama to elicit what they were already familiar with through meditation.

Shinto students were given the kotodama straight away, to chant to get to grips with earth ki etc.

In the Western system there might be chakra meditations, crystals, a 'meet your spirit guide' meditation or some stuff about Angels, at either First or Second Degree.

There will be rules about using symbols in various combinations and rules about when you can, and cannot, use the energy in different situations.

Some Western courses now embrace information coming from Frank Arjava Petter and Hiroshi Doi in terms of 'Gakkai techniques and Reiji ho.

Differences

So the main differences between standard Western Reiki and the original system at Second Degree are that Western Reiki focuses on working on other people almost exclusively, really, using symbols, sometimes in complicated ways, and courses also focus on distant healing.

The original system is free of distant healing and free from symbols and maintains its focus on self-development/spiritual development through the use of meditations or kotodama chanting over an extended period, and through the study of Buddhist sutras.

Treating others is a side-issue and is carried out simply and intuitively, if at all.

The healing ability is a side-effect of the main thrust of the system.

Reiki Master course

Western courses	Original system
Receive attunement(s)	Receive empowerments.
	Receive further spiritual teachings, details not known
	Learn how to empower yourself
	Carry out a series of further self-empowerments
Learn DKM symbol. Learn a variety of non-Reiki symbols and different techniques or meditations from different non-Reiki systems	Be shown the DKM symbol. Learn the empowerment kotodama for use when carrying out self-empowerments
Learn how to attune others	Learn how to empower others, towards the end of your Shinpiden Training
	The goal was 'satori', a flash of insight that changes something in a fundamental way. Satori is something that comes through a long period of meditation, something that you work at by getting rid of your 'baggage'.
	It was an open-ended system for you to carry on your own journey – a lifetime endeavour

Differences

So the main differences between standard Western Reiki and the original system at Shinpiden level are that Western Reiki focuses mainly on attuning other people, and can include working with various symbols and exercises that have come to Reiki from different non-Reiki systems.

In the original system the focus is still on self-development/spiritual development, this time through the use of regular self-empowerments, meditations, and the receiving of spiritual teachings, the details of which aren't know.

We do know, though, that Usui seemed to be passing on the essential teachings of Tendai Buddhism, in a way that could be understood by anyone.

And while achieving 'Mastership' in the Western system seems to be the goal for many people, in the original system this was merely a stepping stone on your journey.

Next, you can see how I put Reiki Evolution courses together: what I included from the original system, what I excluded and what I added to make the courses reasonably compatible with what students learn on standard Hayashi/Takata "Western" Reiki courses...

Creating the Reiki Evolution First Degree course

What I am going to do in this section is to explain how I put together Reiki Evolution courses in terms of what I included of the original system that Mikao Usui taught, what I excluded, what I added, and why.

KEPT	empowerments
KEPT	self-healing
KEPT	precepts
KEPT	mindfulness
KEPT	Kenyoku/Joshin Kokkyu ho on its own and as part of Hatsurei ho because it's a nice sequence, even though not original Usui (came from the 'Gakkai)
ADDED	treating other people to make the courses compatible with Western Reiki
LOST	waka poetry because we don't know what the poems were and because we're not Japanese and couldn't study them in the original language

So we've retained most of the original approach and basically added the treating of others to make the course compatible with what other First Degree practitioners will have learned to do.

But we provide more of a 'loose' system in terms of hand positions, where although we do teach a standard set of positions for students to follow to begin with, they already know that they are going to be moving beyond these through scanning or, ideally, intuitive working.

And our system is free from lots of rules and regulations about what you can and cannot do, because this is unnecessary.

The interval between First and Second Degree

This is a slight sticking point, really, since in the original system students carried out the hara defining exercise and only when they had developed sufficiently in the eyes of their teacher would they have been allowed to move on to Second Degree.

This is a sticking point for me for various reasons:

Firstly, the hara defining exercise is the most tricky of all the Reiki exercises/meditations and I wonder if people would lose interest and perhaps go and train somewhere else if their progression to Second Degree with us was dependent on their carrying out this exercise and being monitored by the teacher over a period of time until the teacher felt that they had done sufficient work to warrant being allowed to take Second Degree.

I thought that the level of commitment required to carry out this exercise would probably be more present in people moving on to RMT level than those who have just completed First Degree, so I have included it on the RMT course.

I wonder how many people get to grips with it even then.

As an aside, students do get to grips with this exercise on my RMT home study course because it's at more of a leisurely pace and they have to do it before I let them move on!

I expect my students to wait for a couple of months, at least, between their First and Second Degree courses, to give them an opportunity to put into practice everything they learned on First Degree.

Creating the Reiki Evolution Second Degree course

Here you can see what I have retained of the original system, what I have left out and what I have added, and why:

KEPT   empowerments
KEPT   experiencing of earth ki and
              heavenly ki, but through the use of
              CKR and SHK symbols
KEPT   oneness, but through use of HSZSN
              and distant healing
KEPT   emphasis on simplicity and intuition
              when treating people
ADDED   more of an emphasis on treating
              others than in original system
ADDED   distant healing to make the course
              compatible with Western Reiki.
LOST   Buddhist sutras and I don't think
              this would be helpful*

* (1) Because we keep on saying that Reiki isn't allied to any Religion, and (2) because we're not Buddhists, don't

155

have the expertise, and it's not our culture; This was 1900s Japan and not everything is transferable.

My teachers and I feel that it was important to carry on teaching the symbols because they are such an important part of Western Reiki and because students may feel 'left out' if they don't have them.

What we're are doing through teaching symbol meditations as a self-healing practice is to echo the original practice of working with earth ki and heavenly ki, but using the symbols as triggers to access these energies, instead of the kotodama.

Trying to teach both kotodama and symbols on a Second Degree course is too much for students to take in, I believe; some people struggle with three Japanese-sounding names, without adding three more slightly different sounds!

Some teachers do teach the kotodama as well as the symbols' names at Second Degree, and it can work for them, but I think it is too confusing at this stage.

Some teachers have chosen to just teach the kotodama at Second Degree, and leave out the Reiki symbols and, while this does indeed echo the original system well, I do not think it is a good idea to leave out of someone's Second Degree training symbols that 99.9% of all Reiki people have been taught.

The interval between Second Degree and Mastership

In the original system, during this pre-Mastery period, students practised 'seated ki breathing' where they connect to earth ki, add heavenly ki, and then allow the energies to find a balance, and once their teacher had decided that the student had advanced sufficiently they would then be allowed to move on to Shinpiden level.

This is really much more suitable to a 'dojo' format, with regular weekly contact between student and teacher, and thus far we have not been teaching the Buddhist-style meditations, or seated ki breathing; I only include them in the RMT manual at the moment.

I expect my students to wait for at least six months between their Second Degree and Master Teacher courses, to give them an opportunity to put into practice everything they learned on Second Degree.

Creating the Reiki Evolution Master Teacher course

Here you can see what I have retained of the original system, what I have left out and what I have added, and why:

KEPT	empowerments
KEPT	self-empowerments
KEPT	empowerment kotodama
KEPT	learning how to perform Reiju
ADDED	Western attunements
ADDED	Kotodama (originally taught at Second Degree)
ADDED	Use of intuition when treating
ADDED	Use of intent when treating
ADDED	Other Western Reiki Master stuff: different symbols, meditations, crystal grids etc, just for the sake of completeness
LOST	further spiritual teachings because we don't know what they were
LOST	further energy exercises beyond energy-ball self-empowerment

So I have included the main themes of the original Shinpiden level, so far as we know what was taught.

I introduce kotodama at RMT level because it would be too complicated to teach them on a Second Degree course as well as the corresponding symbols and symbol names.

The hara defining exercise, Buddhist-style meditations for earth/heaven/oneness are included in the Reiki Evolution Master Teacher manual, as is seated ki breathing.

The emphasis is still on self-development, with the use of kotodama, the hara defining exercise and self-empowerments.

We retain the Western focus on treatments, though give it a strong dose of simplicity through the use of intent and intuition, and for completeness I have included a variety of symbols (for people who like symbols) and the various Western non-Reiki add-ons like crystal grids, antahkaranas, healing attunements and psychic surgery.

I didn't want to censor these things and equally I didn't want to teach them as part of 'Reiki', so they're just there in the manual for students to read about and try for themselves if they feel so inclined.

TEACHING REIKI "REIKI EVOLUTION" STYLE

Introduction

The fact that you have become a Reiki Master/Teacher does not mean that you are now obliged to run courses and teach the general public; you do not need to run courses at all.

Maybe you might decide to pass on the benefits of Reiki to some friends and family members in an informal way and go no further than that, and that's fine.

But if you decide to move on to run formal Reiki training sessions then I have tried to make the process as easy as I can for you.

The first thing to remember about running your own courses is that Reiki is simple and you know far more about the subject than you realise.

When you teach Reiki you are passing on a few practical skills, all skills that you have experience of using yourself.

You have played around with energy and carried out Hatsurei, so you can show someone else how to do the same.

You can help someone to get to grips with self-treatments: you have done loads of self-treatments.

You can show someone how to give a Reiki treatment: you have done it yourself, so you can teach from a solid foundation of practical experience.

This is a complete guide to teaching the Reiki First Degree, Second Degree and the Reiki Master Teacher course in the "Reiki Evolution" style.

In this section you will find, for each course:

1. A course schedule
2. Detailed instructions telling you what to say & do
3. A description of all the practical exercises that your students will carry out during the course

To get a good feel for the two courses I suggest that you immerse yourself in the Reiki Evolution course materials for a good while.

The Reiki Evolution First and Second Degree manuals are comprehensive and detailed and provide you with a good guide to the general thrust and tone and 'slant' of the courses, rooted in the original system that Usui was teaching, but presented in a way that will work in the modern world, echoing the original practices but also reasonably compatible with the 'treatment' emphasis of most Western Reiki courses.

I suggest that you listen to the audio commentary CDs for First and Second Degree several times too, since these focus on the main themes of the courses.

Listening to the Reiki Meditations audio CD will help you to become familiar with what you need to say to talk your students through Hatsurei ho and the Self-treatment meditation on the First Degree course, and Symbol meditations and a Distant healing session.

If you immerse yourself in these materials you will know exactly what your students will have been exposed to, and you can build on that, emphasising the main themes and rooting what you do in the original practices.

What we are doing with these courses is to emphasise what Usui was teaching, and to show how we can follow these basic practices.

The focus is on Reiki as a self-healing, energy-balancing, spiritual-development system, with the treatment of other covered in full to make the course compatible with the 'treatment' focus of most Reiki courses, but with a simple, clutter-free and intuitive approach to treating people.

First Degree

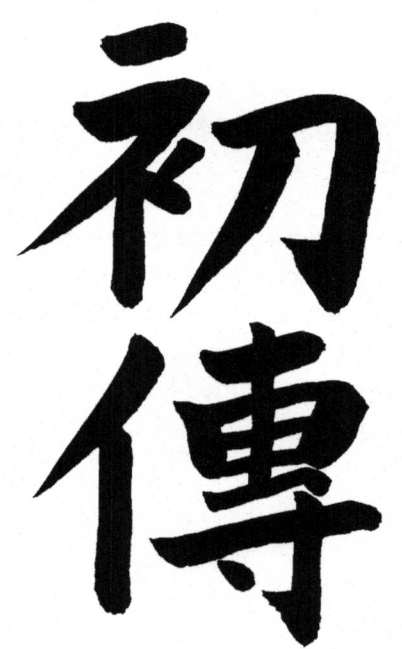

Back to Basics: Reiki First Degree

I thought it would be useful here for me to include a Reiki blog that I have on my web site, where I talk about the essence of Reiki First Degree. Keep these principles in mind, as you read through the detailed instructions that follow it.

This is what I said:

People end up on First Degree courses for many reasons and come from an amazing variety of backgrounds, all attending for their own personal reasons.

Reiki courses in the UK present a whole variety of approaches, some "traditional" Western-style, some more Japanese in content, some wildly different and almost unrecognisable, some free and intuitive, others dogmatic and based on rules about what you should always do and not do. Reiki is taught in so many ways, and students will tend to imagine that the way that they were taught is the way that Reiki is taught and practised by most other Reiki people.

What I have tried to do in this article is to present a simple guide to the essence of First Degree: what it's all about and what we should be doing and thinking about to get the most out of our experience of Reiki at this level. My words are addressed to anyone at First Degree level, or anyone who would like to review the essence of First Degree.

First Degree is all about connecting to the energy, learning to develop your sensitivity to the flow of energy, working on yourself to develop your ability as a channel and to enhance self-healing, and working on other people. There are many approaches to doing these things, and I wanted below to touch on each area and to dispel some myths that may have been passed on.

Connecting to the energy

On your Reiki course you will have received some attunements or some empowerments. Attunements are not standard rituals within the world of Reiki and take many forms, some simpler and some more complex.

They have evolved and changed greatly during their journey from teacher to teacher in the West. There is no "right way" to carry out an attunement and the individual details of a ritual do not matter a great deal. They all work.

Equally, there is no "correct" number of attunements that have to be carried out at First Degree level. The number four is quoted often as being the "correct" number but this has no basis in Reiki's original form, and whether you receive one, two, three or four rituals on your course, that is fine.

On your course you may have received some "empowerments" rather than attunements, though these are less common. The word "empowerment", or "Reiju empowerment", refers to a connection ritual that has come to us from some Japanese sources, and is closer in essence to the empowerment that Mikao Usui conveyed to his students.

Again, there is no correct number of empowerments that has to be carried out. One is enough but it is nice to do more.

What we experience when receiving an attunement or an empowerment will vary a lot. Some people have fireworks and bells and whistles and that's nice for them; other people notice a lot less, very little, or even nothing, and that's fine too.

What we feel when we have an attunement is not a guide to how well it has worked for us. Attunements work, and sometimes we will have a strong experience, but it's not compulsory! Whether we have noticed a lot, or very little, the attunement will have given us what we need.

Since in Mikao Usui's system you would have received empowerments from him again and again, it would be nice if you could echo this practice by receiving further empowerments (or attunements) and perhaps these might be available at your teacher's Reiki shares or get-togethers, if they hold them. But it is possible to receive distant Reiju empowerments and various teachers make them freely available as a regular 'broadcast'.

This is not essential, and your connection to Reiki once given does not fizzle out, but it would be a beneficial practice if you could receive regular empowerments from someone.

Developing your Sensitivity to the energy

People's experience of energy when they first start working with Reiki can vary. Some people notice more than others, particularly in the early stages, and if we perhaps notice less going on in our hands when compared with another student on the course we can become disillusioned to an extent: that little voice in your head says "I know Reiki works for everyone… but it's not going to work for me. I knew it wasn't going to work for me".

Well if this describes your situation then I can say to you that Reiki will work for you, and is working for you, and the vast majority of Reiki people can feel the flow of energy through them in some way, though your particular 'style' of sensing the energy may not involve the more usual heat, fizzing, tingling, pulsing etc. that many people experience.

There are a few Reiki Master/Teachers out there who feel absolutely nothing in their hands, but this is not common, and Reiki is still working for them.

Sensitivity to the flow of energy develops over time, with practice. Some people are lucky enough to be able to feel quite a lot in their hands and in their bodies to begin with, but others have to be patient, trust that Reiki is working for them, and perhaps focus more on the feedback that they receive from the people that they treat, rather than what they feel – or don't feel – in their hands.

It would be worthwhile if all First Degree students spent some time regularly practising feeling energy: between your hands, around your cat or dog or your pot plant or a tree, around someone else's head and shoulders, over someone's supine body, noticing any differences in the sensation in your hands as you move your hands from one place to another.

Don't expect to experience a particular thing or a particular intensity of feeling. Be neutral and simply notice what experience you have and how that experience might change from one area to another.

On some First Degree courses this process will be taught as "scanning", where you hover your hands over the recipient's body, drift your hands from one place to another, and notice any areas which are drawing more energy. This can provide some useful information in terms of suggesting additional or alternative hand-positions to use when you treat, and can suggest areas where you are going to spend longer when you treat.

Working on yourself

It is vital that after going on a First Degree course you establish a regular routine of working on yourself in order to develop your fledgling ability as a channel and to obtain the benefits that Reiki can provide in terms of balancing your life and self-healing.

Most people decide to learn Reiki because they are looking for some personal benefits as well as looking to help other people, and the way to get the most out of the Reiki system is to work on yourself regularly.

On your First Degree course you will have been taught a self-treatment method, perhaps a Japanese-style meditation but more likely the Western "hands-on" self-treatment method. You will most likely have been given a set of hand-positions to use, but please remember that these positions are not set in stone and, particularly if some of the hand positions are quite uncomfortable to use in practice, you will develop your own style.

It is fine to change the hand positions based on what feels right from one self-treatment to another, and you should do what feels appropriate. There is no "correct" set of positions that you have to use, and each hand-position does not have to be held for a particular period of time. Treat for however long you have time for, and however long feels right for each hand-position you decide to use.

Many people are taught that they have to do a "21 day self-treat", and some people have the impression that they then do not need to self-treat any more. The "21 day" period has no real basis, and I can say that you ought to be thinking in terms of working on yourself long-term.

To gain the greatest benefits from this wonderful system you need to persevere and make working with energy a permanent feature of your life with Reiki, a basic background practice, the effects of which will build up cumulatively as you continue to work with the energy.

You may have been taught a series of energy exercises and meditations called "Hatsurei ho" which comes from Japanese Reiki, and I can commend this practice to you. It is a wonderful way of grounding, balancing, and enhancing you ability as a channel, and should be a regular part of your Reiki routine.

Treating other people

First Degree is also about starting to work on other people, a process which also benefits the giver, so plus points all round really! A few students may have been taught not to treat others at First Degree, or for a particular prescribed period, but this is an unnecessary restriction and Reiki can be shared with other people straight away.

There are many different approaches to treating others, and we should not get bogged down with too many rules and regulations about how we 'must' proceed.

Reiki can be approached in quite a regimented way in some lineages, and students may worry that if they are not remembering all the stages that they 'have' to carry out then they will not be carrying out the treatment properly. This is an unnecessary worry because treating other people is simple.

So here is a simple approach that you can use: close your eyes, maybe put your hands in the prayer position, and take a few long deep breaths to calm you and still your mind.

You should have in mind that the energy you will channel should be for the highest good of the recipient, but there is no particular form of words that you need to use when commencing your treatment.

Now we are going to focus your attention on connecting to the energy. Imagine that energy is flooding down to you from above, flooding through your crown, through the centre of your body, down to your Dantien (an energy centre two fingerbreadths below your tummy button and 1/3rd of the way into your body). Imagine the energy building up and intensifying there. You are filling with energy.

Now direct your attention towards the recipient and imagine that you are merging with them, becoming one with them. Feel compassion and enjoy the moment.

You may now begin your treatment, and maybe it would be nice to rest your hands on their shoulders for a while, to connect to them and to get the energy flowing. What hand positions you use will vary depending on what you were taught – there are many variations – and they are all variations on a theme, a way of firing the energy from lots of different directions to give it the best chance of getting to where it needs to go.

Hand-positions for treating others are not set in stone and do not have to be followed slavishly.

They are just there as a set of guidelines to follow to build your confidence when treating others, and with time and practice you will start to leave behind these basic instructions and gear any treatment towards the needs of the recipient on that occasion, perhaps based on what you picked up when you were 'scanning' and perhaps based on intuitive impressions, where you feel drawn to a particular area of the body.

Don't try and work out 'why' you have felt drawn to a particular area of the body: just accept your impression and go with it.

Reiki is basically a hands-on treatment method, though for reasons of comfort and propriety you will choose to hover your hands over the recipient in some areas rather than resting on the body.

I do not plaster my hands over the recipient's face or throat, for example, because I think that this is uncomfortable and unsettling for the person you are working on.

You do not have to hover your hands for every hand position, as some people are taught, and equally you do not have to keep at least one hand in physical contact with the recipient's body at all times, for fear of 'losing' your connection: your connection to the recipient is a state of mind, and where your hands are is irrelevant!

As you treat, you should aim to feel yourself merging with the energy, becoming one with the energy, to imagine yourself disappearing into the energy, and this can give you a quite blissful experience.

Your mind may wander, particularly in the early stages of your Reiki practice, but you do not need to worry about this. If you notice thoughts intruding, pay them no attention; let them drift on like clouds.

If you make a big effort to try and get rid of your thoughts then you will have in your head the original thoughts and then all the new thoughts about getting rid of the first lot of thoughts… you have made things worse! Just bring your attention gently back to the recipient, to the energy, feel yourself disappearing into the energy, merging with the recipient, and let the energy flow; your treatment can become a wonderful meditation.

It is not acceptable to chat to other people while giving a Reiki treatment.

If you want to be an effective channel for the energy then you need to direct your attention to the work at hand and make sure you are not unduly distracted. For this reason, conversation between yourself and the recipient should be restricted.

Reiki works best of you are still and focused, merging with the energy, in a gentle meditative state. Developing this state takes practice and you can't do it properly if you are chatting.

You do not need to stay for a particular set amount of time for each hand position.

Though it would be probably be best to stay for a few minutes in each position, if in a particular hand position you feel a lot of energy coming through your hands then you can stay in that position for longer – sometimes a lot longer – until the sensation subsides and you can then move onto the next area.

Your hands can guide you.

Work from the head and shoulders, down the length of the body, and it is nice to finish with the ankles.

Many people are taught to smooth down the energy field at the end of a session, and that is a nice thing to do, but remember that you do not have to follow any rituals slavishly, particularly in terms of any sort of 'closing' ritual; you do not need to touch the ground, you do not need to say a particular set of words, you do not need to visualise anything in particular, and you do not need to make any 'set' movements of your hands or body.

The Reiki Precepts

On your First Degree course you will have been introduced to the Reiki Precepts, or Reiki Principles, Mikao Usui's "rules to live by".

Just in case you have been given a slightly distorted version of the precepts, here is a more accurate translation:

> *The secret of inviting happiness through many blessings*
> *The spiritual medicine for all illness*
>
> *For today only: Do not anger; Do not worry*
> *Be humble*
> *Be honest in your dealings with people*

Be compassionate to yourself and others

Do gassho every morning and evening

Keep in your mind and recite

The founder, Usui Mikao

Any reference to 'honouring your elders, parents and teachers' is a later addition to the list, and is not what Mikao Usui taught.

The precepts were the hub of the whole system, and it is said that as much spiritual development can come through following the precepts in your daily life as would come from any energy work, so they are important.

If we can try to focus on living in the moment, not forever dwelling on the past or worrying about the future (fear is a distraction), if we can remind ourselves of the many blessings we have in our lives, if we can forgive ourselves for not being perfect and if we can see things from another's point of view, if we can be compassionate towards ourselves as well as others, then we have gone a long way towards achieving a liberating sense of serenity and contentment. This is not something to be achieved overnight, of course: it is a work-in-progress.

Finally

Reiki has the potential to make an amazing, positive difference to you and the people around you. Remember that Reiki is simplicity itself, and by taking some steps to work on yourself regularly, and share Reiki with the people close to you, you are embarking on a very special journey.

How far you travel on that journey is governed by how many steps you take.

Course Schedule: First Degree

Here you can see a basic structure for your Reiki First Degree course, showing what to cover in the morning and afternoon session.

The course is held on a single day and assumes that the student has spent some time before the course reading the course manual and listening to the course audio CDs.

That way, they know a lot about what they are going to be doing on the course and, rather then spending a lot of time as a teacher sitting telling them stuff that they could have read about beforehand, you can concentrate on the practical stuff: helping them to work with energy for their own benefit and to help other people.

So the course is all about summarising and recapping things that the student is already familiar, and putting everything into practice.

Students arrive at 9.30am, starting the course at 10am the latest. Break for lunch, say 45 minutes. Afternoon session starts by 2pm. Finish 5pm – 5.30pm latest

Introduction
Ask students to talk for a little about why they are on a Reiki course
Let them know about the possible clear-out
Talk a little bit about the original system and what they are going to do today
Emphasise the Reiki precepts and Usui's focus on mindfulness, for them to investigate

Reiju empowerment # 1
Feedback on their experiences

Introduce students to working with energy
Feeling energy between the hands
Feeling energy on someone else's hands
Feeling/scanning energy field around head/shoulders

Reiju empowerment # 2
Feedback on their experiences

Talk about importance of daily energy exercises
Demonstrate Hatsurei
Talk them through the whole Hatsurei ho, leading to ...

Reiju empowerment # 3
Feedback on their experiences

Talk about self-treatment methods, and advantages of self-treatment meditation
Demonstrate Self-treatment meditation
Talk them through the Usui self-treatment meditation

[LUNCH]

Talk about treating others
Different treatment approaches: short blasts,
head/shoulders, full treatments
Simple scheme to get things going: affirm, connect,
build, merge, flow
Feeling the energy field and scanning
Demonstrate some hand positions
Smoothing down the energy field and disconnecting

Treating others
Students carry out a full treatment on each other. Two
treatment tables will be needed for four students.

Students start with feeling the energy field/scanning.
Encourage them.
Then talk the students through each stage/hand
position.

At the end of each treatment obtain feedback from the
treater and the recipient

Conclusion
Tell them how well they have done, remind them of the
main themes of the course, and remind them of their
homework

Points to make on the First Degree course

These are some notes, based on the sort of points that I have made on my courses, for information and guidance. I do not expect you to say the same things as me, and I do not expect you to only make these points, but the following notes give you an idea of some of the things that could be said.

The important thing is to keep things simple, remind students of the basic practices of the original system as they progress through the course, and to emphasise personal responsibility: they need to go away and do the work regularly to obtain the benefits that are available through Reiki.

Morning session

Your Introduction

Welcome to Reiki First Degree, the first part of a two-part basic course in Reiki.

First Degree stands alone; you are not obliged to go on to Second Degree level, but most people do. You've already had a chance to go through the course manual and listen to the audio CD, so you already know a lot about Reiki; today's course is mainly practical. In effect this is a 2 ½ day course: you have spent about a day and a half working with the manual and audio CD, and now we do the practical part of the course.

You've already seen the schedule for today, but I'll just run through the things that we are going to be doing…

(1)

During the morning you will be receiving three Japanese empowerments.

The strange thing about Reiki is that while you can find out about Reiki by reading books or looking on the Internet, you can't actually do Reiki until you have been tuned in by a Reiki Master (which just means teacher).

We'll be going through three connection rituals that will tune you in to the energy.

Reiki works for everyone: you haven't got to be a massively spiritual person, you don't even have to believe in Reiki… you just need to go on a course and be attuned and it will work for you.

(2)

Morning is broken into three sections, each one starting with an empowerment.

Section One

We will carry out some exercises where you'll start to experience your own energy, and other people's.

Section Two

You'll learn a series of energy exercises / meditations / visualisations that you can use every day to help make you a progressively stronger clearer channel for Reiki.

Section Three

We'll finish the morning by talking a little about self-treatments and we'll practice a self-treatment meditation that you've already been reading about.

… so the morning focuses on getting you used to experiencing energy, and background practices that you can use every day to help make you a stronger channel for Reiki and to focus the energy on yourself for self-balancing.

One of the wonderful things about Reiki is that you can share the energy with other people by way of giving treatments, so in the afternoon we'll talk about treatments, I'll demonstrate some hand positions that you can use, show you how to do "scanning" and you'll split into pairs and treat each other… so by the end of the afternoon you will have given a full treatment and received a full treatment, and you'll be ready to unleash yourself on unsuspecting friends and family members!

Reiki is a hand-on practical subject, so once you've finished today's course you'll need to work with the energy regularly, on yourself and on others.

Their Introductions

Ask students to explain what on earth they're doing here / how they have ended up learning Reiki… not 45 minutes describing their entire life and all the events that led them to being here today, but just a few minutes giving us an idea of how you've ended up here.

[Take the opportunity to pick up on things they have said to make a few interesting points about Reiki.]

"The Warning"

Remind them that once you've been attuned to Reiki, the energy can get to you all the time, and it will start to bring things into balance.

Part of bringing things into balance involves getting rid of stuff, ditching things that you can do without. So over the next few weeks you might feel tiredness, you might have headaches or aches and pains, you might have some emotional ups and downs, you might feel dissatisfied with everyone and everything: doubting your job, doubting your relationship... looking at various aspects of your life and working out what your real priorities are.

So you might be cursing me in a week's time, or you might be absolutely fine!

It is not possible in an individual case to predict whether you are going to have a strong reaction or not, but for most people it's no great shakes, and Reiki doesn't seem to give people stuff that they can't handle.

The Original System

Remind them that what Usui was teaching was a simple self-healing and spiritual development system that might occasionally have been used to treat other people, which has 'morphed' over time into something that is presented to the world as a sort of complementary therapy.

Our courses are trying to get to back to the focus of the original practice, while still including a treatment emphasis (so that these courses are reasonably compatible with the general run of Western-style Reiki courses), and presenting the original practices in a way that will work for a modern Western audience.
Usui's system consisted of:

1. Following a set of precepts and practising mindfulness
2. Receiving spiritual empowerments on a regular basis
3. Carrying out simple energy exercises each day
4. Performing some sort of self-treatment

The precepts were the very foundation of the system, and as much development was said to be possible through following the precepts as would come through carrying out the energy work. We can learn to live the precepts through considering them in turn and deciding for ourselves how they impinge on your behaviour, reactions and relationships.

It would be useful if the student spent some time reading about mindfulness and trying to make this a part of their life.

We provide Reiju empowerments in person on this course, and then at a distance each week on Mondays, for students to tune into.

The course will equip the student to carry out both daily energy exercises and self-treatments, with an audio CD to talk the student through the exercises.

And we cover the treatment of others fully, so that the course is compatible with the 'treatment' focus of most Reiki courses.

Giving the First Empowerment

I tell them that I am not going to suggest to them what they might notice when receiving an empowerment, because I don't want to put ideas into their head.

I tell them that they will be sitting quietly with their hands resting in their laps, listening to the music and feeling themselves becoming peaceful and relaxed. When it is their turn to receive their empowerment I will rest my hand on their shoulder, which is a cue for them to bring their hands into the prayer position.

I will carry out their empowerment, which does not involve touching them or making contact with them, and when the empowerment is over I'll bring their hands back down into their lap.

Then they will wait quietly with their eyes closed until I have finished with everyone else, and then I'll bring them all back together.

… and then we'll see what they noticed, not because I'm looking for a particular thing, but because it's nice to see how experiences vary from one person to another.

An important point to make is that what you feel when you receive an empowerment is no guide to how well it has worked. People's experiences vary greatly from one person to another.

If you read books about Reiki then everyone seems to be having religious ecstasy, but it doesn't really work quite like that in practice. It seems to follow a 'standard distribution curve'.

On one end of the scale you have the people who are having fireworks, bells and whistles, on the other end are the people who just feel a bit relaxed and not much more than that… and most people are in the middle, feeling something but without it being a big earth-shattering experience.

Unfortunately, what happens sometimes is that there will be a group of people: three talking animatedly about all the interesting things they have noticed and one poor soul thinking "Hmmmn, well it obviously hasn't worked for me".

What you feel when you have an empowerment is not a guide as to how well it has worked for you. Some people seem to naturally notice a lot more happening than others. Reiki works for everyone.

Introducing them to energy

Reiki is all about energy, and the idea of energy may seem a little strange at first.

Energy is all around you, though. Your body is composed of it, energy flows through you, energy surrounds you, it is right under your nose. But in the West we don't even spend five minutes trying to experience the energy.

When we do change our focus, when we change what we are focusing our attention on, we can start to experience energy really easily.

[I go through three exercises with the students (see schedule above): feeling the energy between their hands, feeling the energy field around someone else's palm, and feeling the energy field/scanning the head/shoulders of someone sitting in a chair in front of them.

For each exercise I get everyone to describe their sensations and experiences, and the first exercise I might do a couple of times if not everyone 'gets it' the first time. They usually do.]

[For the third exercise I get them to not just feel the energy field but to see if they can find areas where the feeling changes in some way: heat, fizzing, buzzing, pulsing, coolness, a breeze blowing under their hand, magnetic pulsing. If they do feel some change then they move away from that area, and drift back again to see if the distinctive sensation repeats. They see if they can find a number of areas where the feeling is different in some way.]

[At the end of this session I encourage them by saying that despite this being the first time they've done anything like this, they are already sensitive enough to the energy to not just be able to feel the energy field but to be able to feel variations in the flow of energy... and that we will be doing more work on that in the afternoon when they practise scanning each other on the treatment tables.]

Hatsurei ho

Hatsurei is a series of energy exercises that you can do every day. You do Hatsurei for these reasons:

1. Clear and cleanse your energy system
2. Help to move your energy system more into a state of balance
3. Help to ground you
4. Help to build up your personal energy reserves
5. Develop your ability as a channel for Reiki
6. Help to develop your sensitivity to the flow of energy
7. Help to develop your intuitive side

Hatsurei consists of two introductory stages and three meditations/visualisations, some of which involve using the Tanden.

The Tanden is energy centre found two finger-breadths below your tummy button and a third of the way into your body. It is seen as the focus of personal power, your personal energy store, and it turns up in energy cultivation techniques like tai chi and qi gong: you go through the graceful movements to build up your reserves of chi, and you store this new chi in your Tanden

In martial arts you might draw down energy from the sun and concentrate it in your Tanden before sparring with someone.

The Tanden is also seen as the centre of your universe, the centre of you being, the place where your soul resides, the centre of your creativity and intuition.

So when you perform Japanese calligraphy you focus your attention on your Tanden, when you do Ikebana (flower arranging) you focus your attention on your Tanden, and even when you perform the Tea Ceremony.

In Hatsurei we will be imagining that energy or light is passing into our Tanden and then moving off elsewhere.

Now if this the first time you have done anything like this then it is highly likely that you won't feel anything happening in your Tanden. This may be the first time that you have even considered a point two fingerbreadths below your tummy button and a third of the way into your body!

After a few weeks or maybe months of practice, you may start to notice a dull fizzy warmth or heaviness in that area. But because Reiki follows your thoughts, it follows your focus, if you imagine energy moving to your Tanden then it will, and it is quite a separate thing as to whether you can actually feel it happening.

Self-treatments

You've already seen from the manual that there are various ways of carrying out self-treatments. For most of Reiki's history in the West people have treated themselves by putting their hands on themselves.

I think that most people who self-treat in that way will do it when they go to bed at night: you don't need a treatment couch, you are already horizontal, without too many distractions... and many people use Reiki self-treatments as a way of getting off to sleep at night.

Disadvantages are that you can easily fall asleep when you're doing it, some of the hand positions on the head can be quite uncomfortable to hold for any amount of time, and it's not really suitable to use in public places! If you're a passenger on a train then you're going to attract a lot of attention and you might whack someone in the head as you try to hold some of the hand positions!

But it can be lovely to sit with your hands resting on the heart and solar plexus, and after a while – as you become more sensitive to the energy – you can feel something like "Ralgex" deep penetrating right to the centre of you.

You could sit like this in the evening while watching television, and if you are chatting to someone then the energy won't come through as strongly as if you were just still and focused on what you were doing... but it would still come through to an extent.

But from Usui's surviving students has come a way of self-treating based on visualising: a self-treatment meditation.

What you do is to imagine that a carbon copy of you is sitting there on the floor in front of you, and in your mind's eye you imagine that you are treating that imaginary you, energy flooding out of your hands into a number of standard positions on the head, which you have already been reading about in your manual.

You might want to try imagining yourself being treated by the carbon copy, or seeing yourself being treated by some disembodied hands.

Or perhaps don't visualise anything, and simply allow your attention to rest or to dwell on those areas of your head. The positions are [demonstrate them]:

- Hovering your hands in front of the forehead, by the hair line
- Hands by the temples, the sides of the head
- Cupping your hands round the back of the head and resting on the forehead
- Hands on the back of the neck and the base of the skull
- Hands hovering above the crown

Now as you do this you may notice that you have a feeling of there being 'hands' by your real head, and you may find it easier to have the carbon copy of you standing there behind you, treating the 'real' you.

Experiment with this as we go through the meditation to see what feels best for you.

What makes this way of self-treating so exciting is that it is so versatile: you can now treat yourself any time you can just sit down for a while with your eyes closed, even for a few minutes.

So if you are a passenger on a train or in a car, or at work during a ten-minute break, you can self-treat... which makes it a lot more likely that you will self-treat regularly.

You should experiment and become familiar with all types of self-treatment.

Conclusion to the Morning

This morning has focused on introducing you to energy
– your own energy and other people's – and we have
learned background practices that will make you a
strong clear channel for the energy and which will
enhance the beneficial effects that Reiki has on you.
You have come on this course because you want to get
some benefit out of Reiki, and the way to do that is to
work with the energy regularly... so my prescription for
success with Reiki is to carry out Hatsurei every day –
start your day with Hatsurei! – and to self-treat ideally
every day.

Afternoon session

Giving Reiki treatments

What I am going to be showing you is a 'formal' hour-long Reiki treatment. If you go to a Reiki practitioner for a treatment then you'll end up having a treatment lasting for about 50 minutes / 1 ¼ hours. But just because I am showing you a full treatment doesn't mean that you are always obliged to spend an hour treating someone.

If someone has a pain in their knee, then sit yourselves down on the floor next to them and plonk your hands on their knee for 10 minutes.

If someone has a headache then sit them in a chair and treat their head and shoulders for 15-20 minutes.

Go with what time you have available... so you can give 'short blasts' of Reiki, you can give head and shoulder treatments, and you can give full treatments. The important thing is to get the hands-on practice.

[Someone gets onto the treatment table as a guinea pig] You've already been reading the manual and listening to the audio CD where I talk about treating others, so I'm only going to quickly recap the main points.

There is a simple scheme that you can follow whenever you work on someone, to get things going. There are five things to do: affirm, connect, build, merge, flow.

Affirm

When we treat someone we are neutral. We have no expectations. We are not pushing for a particular end result. We do not do Reiki to get rid of someone's headache or to resolve a particular condition… we just let the energy do whatever is right for that person. To remind ourselves of this we can bring our hands into the prayer position, take a few deep breaths to still our mind, and say to ourselves that we dedicate the treatment to the person's 'highest good' or 'highest healing good'.

Connect

Now we 'connect' to Reiki. Of course you are always connected, so what we do here is to focus our attention on our connection to the energy. You can keep your hands in the prayer position (probably the easiest way), you can hold your hands out to the sides, or you can 'connect' using the hand position from Hatsurei. Imagine energy is passing down to you from above, flooding through your crown and passing down to your Tanden.

Build

When we do Reiki we work from the Tanden. We focus on the Tanden when we practise Hatsurei, we can focus on the Tanden when we self-treat, and we work from the Tanden when we treat other people. It is our energy store, the centre of our being and the place where our intuition resides. So as the energy flows down to us, we imagine that the energy builds and builds in the Tanden, getting stronger and stronger.

Merge

Now we feel ourselves merging with the energy that is flowing down to us, we can imagine ourselves disappearing into the energy, becoming one with the energy. We merge with the person on the table in front of us. There is no them, there is no us, we become one.

Flow

And finally, we allow the energy to flow, drawn through us according to the need of the recipient, We stand aside and do not direct the energy. We just allow it to flow.

Feeling the energy field

Not everyone can do this, but it's a useful thing to do if you can do it. You won't feel something on everyone you practise on, and you won't necessarily feel something over all of a person's body, but it's a good exercise to help build up your sensitivity to the energy and it can give you some useful information.

Just like earlier on when we were feeling the energy field around the head and shoulders, now we slowly bounce our hands down until we make contact with that layer of energy, or get an impression that our hands are resting on the layer of the energy.

Bounce your hands on that surface a few times to convince yourself that it's definitely there.

Now move on to feel the energy field over an adjacent part of the body, moving up towards the head and down towards the feet. Is the energy field about the same distance away from the body, or are there areas where it seems closer?

If the energy field is closer then it gives you an idea of general relative depletion in that area and you will probably spend a bit more time working on that area when you treat.

Scanning

As you feel the energy field – just like this morning – you may notice that the feeling that you get in some areas is more intense, or you get a distinctive feeling in some places. This is what we look for when we do 'scanning', and it is easier to this one-handed.

Just hover your hand over the person – you don't need to rest your hand on the layer of energy: you are just hovering your hand in a comfortable position over them. Now let your hand drift and focus your attention on the surface of your palm and fingers.

Notice if there are areas where more energy is coming through. You might notice, heat, fizzing/buzzing, pulsing/throbbing, coldness, a breeze blowing under your hand. Look for areas where things feel more intense.

If you find some areas, drift away again; drift back again to see if the sensation repeats each time you go there.

Compare symmetrical areas of the body: hips, knees, and ankles. Does one side feel more intense that the other? Joints are good places to practice on: quite often you'll feel a little 'dzzzt', a little spike of energy as you move past the ankle, the knee, maybe the hip.

People use their joints all the time, they're damaged all the time, and Reiki rushes in to support natural healing.

People scan to 'get the lie of the land' and work out where they're going to be spending more time during the treatment.

Scanning can also suggest extra hand positions too: if you notice that one area of the body is drawing lots of energy and it isn't covered by one of the standard hand positions, then just add an extra hand position or alter your hand positions to make sure that you rest your hands on all the areas that are drawing most energy.

Your hands can also tell you how long to stay in each hand position.

Although you usually hold each position for 3, 4, 5 minutes, if there loads of energy coming through and your hands are going like crazy, then just stay there for a lot longer. After a while the sensations will subside and you know it's ok to move on to the next area.

I am going to be showing you a set of hand positions to use to begin with, but they're not set in stone at all.

They're just guidelines, some instructions to follow to begin with, and with practice you'll start to go more freestyle, and alter your hand positions for each person you work on

One way of moving beyond the standard positions is through scanning, where you may notice some areas that need to be treated that aren't covered by the standard hand positions.

Another way of modifying your hand positions is through intuition: you may notice that you are strangely 'drawn' to as particular area.

Well, don't analyse it, just go with it and treat that area. On the Second Degree course we'll learn a specific technique where you deliberately make yourself open to the intuitive side of things so that the energy guides your hands, rather like having your hands pulled by invisible magnets to the right places to treat.

[I demonstrate the hand positions: shoulders, temples, crown, back of head, front of face, throat, heart/solar plexus, navel, hips, upper leg, knees, ankles.]

Demonstrating treatment hand positions

During the demonstration I make these sorts of points…

Shoulders

Keep your fingers reasonably together as you treat.
When you first make contact with someone, some Reiki
people will say "Reiki On!" silently to themselves, just a
little ritual that says "OK, I'm doing Reiki now, let's be in
the best state of mind for doing Reiki…".

While most hand positions get held for 3,4,5 minutes, I
tend to hold the shoulders for about 10 minutes at the
start of the treatment. It works really well to make people
calm, peaceful, relaxed, getting rid of all their stress and
tension… some people can even be half way to being
fast asleep before you even leave the shoulders
(particularly men!).

Face positions

I tend not to touch the face when I'm treating. They've
just got nice and relaxed and dreamy and then you're
plastering your hands all over their face, which is quite
disruptive. So I keep my hands away from the face.
Reiki works just as well with your hands away from the
body (though Reiki is basically a hands-on therapy).

Throat

You don't grab them by the throat because that wouldn't be relaxing at all! Just cup your hands near to their throat. If there's a lot of energy going into the throat then they cold have a sore throat coming, but quite often it can tie in with the communication side of things, if they're holding back, not expressing themselves, not saying the things that they need to to the people close to them… that can show as a lot of energy going into the throat area.

Heart / Solar Plexus

When we spoke about treating ourselves hands-on, this morning, I spoke about treating the heart and solar plexus at the same time. Well you can do that when you treat another person too. If you're treating a man then you can just rest both hands down; if you're treating a lady then you'd hover your hand over the heart area, with the centre of your palm over the midline of the body: it's the heart energy centre that you're aiming for, not the anatomical heart.

Navel

What you mustn't do when you treat someone is to get yourself into the frame of mind where you think that every 'hotspot' you find is some dread disease that the person doesn't know about yet, and they go away a real hypochondriac because you have said "well there's something going on there, and there, and there's definitely something going on there…".

Reiki rushes in to support very ordinary, boring physiological processes, so if you've had a big lunch then Reiki will rush into the stomach to support digestion; it doesn't mean that they have a stomach ulcer! If you exercise, or go to the gym, then there's going to be a lot going on in the joints: knees and ankles, maybe hips; when you exercise you damage the joints, rip muscle fibres, and they are repaired routinely, and Reiki will rush in to support that. It doesn't mean that they have arthritis.

In the lower abdomen there's a lot more going on in women than in men; you can even work out which side is ovulating based on how much energy is going in on one side rather than the other… it doesn't mean that they have an ovarian cyst.

So all you can say when you find a hotspot, or fizzy area, is that Reiki is rushing in to bring things into balance. You may not know what is being dealt with, but you don't need to.

In some areas it is fairly clear: for example they have had a cartilage operation and loads of energy is rushing into their knee, but when you get to the torso it can get more complicated: in Traditional Chinese Medicine thoughts and emotional states are said to be held in different organs, so your liver holds the emotion of anger and the ability to plan, the gall bladder holds the ability to make decisions, the lungs hold grief, the spleen holds the ability to be able to sift and sort ideas.

So someone can come for a Reiki treatment and not tell you what the problem is, and it won't make any difference to the quality of the treatment you give them, because you simply follow the flow of energy and Reiki gives them what they need on that occasion.

Hips

The precise arrangement and angle of your hands isn't vital. Just find a position that feels comfortable for you.

Knees

If it feels like there is more energy going into one knee than the other, then spend some time with both hands resting on one knee to boost the healing effect.

Ankles

Quite a nice position to finish with. It seems to help bring people back into the land of the living, start to ground them.

Finishing the treatment

Firstly, since you've spent the last hour messing around with their energy field and making it all ruffled, it's nice to smooth things down, so make a number of sweeps from the crown towards the ankles with the intention – and intention is the important thing here – that you are smoothing the energy field down all the way round the body, 360 degrees.

I imagine that there is an invisible hula hoop moving along the length of the body, rather like a magician who's just levitated someone and they're showing that there are no wires.

And when you're happy with that then you do something to say "I've disconnected". You tuned yourself in at the beginning, and now at the end you disconnect yourself.

And the treatment is over.

Conclusion to the day

So now you are ready to unleash yourself on unsuspecting friends and family members!

Reiki is a hands-on practical subject so it is important to get the hands-on practice. Rope people in, tell them that you've learned a Japanese stress-reduction technique and that at the end of a treatment they'll feel so calm, contented, serene... most people won't say "no" to that, and you will be amazed by what happens.

Do short blasts for 5 minutes, 15-20 minutes on their head and shoulders, and full sessions too. It's only when you start treating other people that you really realise what Reiki can do, and that will help build your confidence.

Reiki is simple and safe, so you can't mess up a treatment and leave a person worse off, and you get the benefit of the energy when you treat too, so it's plus points all round.

But remember that Reiki is primarily a way of benefiting yourself through regular practice. You need to practise Hatsurei every day and give yourself self-treatments regularly.

You have a couple of tracks on your "Reiki Meditations" audio CD that talk you through Hatsurei and the self-treatment meditation, so you don't have to remember the stages: just flip on the CD and follow the instructions. You don't even need to worry about how long you're taking with each stage.

You know that the precepts are a very important part of Usui's system, so focus on them, think about them, decide how they apply to your life, and work towards echoing these principles in your daily life.

Reiki 1 Practical Exercises

On the morning of the Reiki1 course I go through some exercises with the students to introduce them to the idea of energy, to try and make things more tangible for them, to make the idea of energy seem real.

Here are some notes from my Reiki1 manual, which give you some idea of the things that I get my students to do.

I don't do these three exercises on every course.

"Reiki is all about energy, and the idea of energy may seem a little strange at first. Energy is all around you, though. Your body is composed of it, energy flows through you, energy surrounds you, it is right under your nose. But in the West we don't even spend five minutes trying to experience the energy. When we do change our focus, when we change what we are focusing our attention on, we can start to experience energy."

Feel Energy Between your Hands

Rub your hands together for half a minute, rather like you are warming your hands up after being out in the cold. Now hold your hands out in front of you, shoulder width apart, with your palms facing each other, rather like you were holding the sides of a very large ball.

Now slowly 'bounce' your hands together until you have an impression that there is something tangible between your hands. You may feel something squashy like a marshmallow, a balloon or a rubber ball; you may feel a surface, a layer, some resistance, some magnetic repulsion… some 'thing' that your hands are resting on that prevents them from touching.

Now obviously you can move your hands all the way together, but with a few attempts most people can feel something between their hands that they can rest their hands on, bounce their hands against. Sometimes you can find a position where your hands don't want to come any closer, but equally they don't want to move away from each other either, a position of balance.

You are feeling your energy field. You have always been able to do this. It has always been right there in front of you. To experience it you have simply changed your focus.

Feel Energy on a Partner's Hand

You will need someone to do this exercise with you. Sit fairly near to each other.

Both of you should rub your hands together for half a minute, rather like you are warming your hands up after being out in the cold.

Now hold one hand out in front of you, at shoulder height, with your palm facing your partner's palm, rather like you were about to push his/her hand away from you.

Now slowly 'bounce' your hands together until you have an impression that there is something tangible between your hands.

You may feel something squashy like a marshmallow, a balloon or a rubber ball; you may feel a surface, a layer, some resistance, some magnetic repulsion… some 'thing' that your hands are resting on that prevents them from touching.

See if you can agree between yourselves about the point where you can both feel that 'contact', that layer or surface, that magnetic repulsion or resistance.

Now one person should keep their hand still while the other person slowly moves their hand vertically up and

down, from side to side, and slowly towards and away from their partner's palm.
How does this feel? What sensations are you experiencing? How do the sensations change?

Now swap over.

The person whose hand was moving should now keep their hand still, and the other person moves their hand around (as described above). Again, how does this feel?

What sensations are you experiencing? How do the sensations change? Now both move your hands, together and away from each other. How does this feel? What sensations are you experiencing? How do the sensations change?

You are feeling the other person's energy field, and you are feeling the reaction of your energy field top the other person's energy field.

You have always been able to do this. It has always been right there in front of you. To experience this you have simply changed your focus.

Feel Energy on a Partner's Head & Shoulders

You will need someone to do this exercise with you.

One person sits in a dining chair and closes their eyes. They are the 'guinea pig' and just sit there throughout the exercise. The other person stands behind them.

The person standing up starts with their hands raised, hovering about 12" (30cm) above the subject's head, palms down. Now bring your hands slowly down, bouncing them down until you feel that your hands are resting on the subject's energy field.

Now move your hands away again and 'bounce' them down onto an adjacent area above the head.

Feel the energy field over different parts of the subject's head, the forehead, the back of the head and the temples.

Is the energy field the same distance away all round the head? Does it feel the same in all places? Feel the energy field over the shoulders, above, behind and in front. How does the energy field feel here?

Second Degree

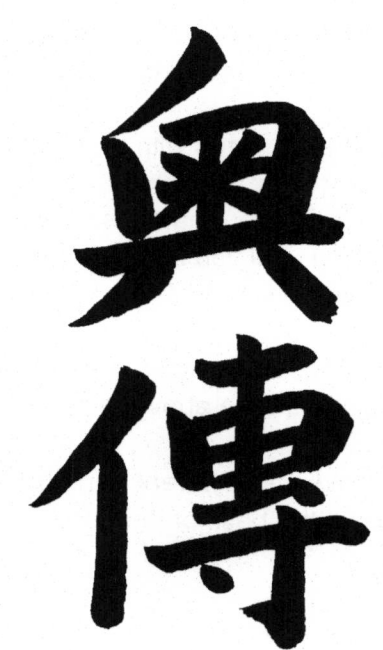

Back to Basics: Reiki Second Degree

I thought it would be useful here for me to include a Reiki blog that I have on my web site, where I talk about the essence of Reiki Second Degree. Keep these principles in mind, as you read through the detailed instructions that follow it.

This is what I said:

People learn Reiki for many reasons and come from an amazing variety of backgrounds, all attending for their own personal reasons. Reiki courses in the UK present a whole variety of approaches, some "traditional" Western-style, some more Japanese in content, some wildly different and almost unrecognisable, some free and intuitive, others dogmatic and based on rules about what you should always do and not do.

Reiki is taught in so many ways, and students will tend to imagine that the way that they were taught is the way that Reiki is taught and practised by most other Reiki people.

What I have tried to do in this article is to present a simple guide to what in my view is the essence of Second Degree: what it's all about and what we should be doing and thinking about to get the most out of our experience of Reiki at this level.

My words are addressed to anyone at Second Degree level, or anyone who would like to review the essence of Second Degree.

The first thing I want to say is that there should usually be an interval of a couple of months or so between First and Second Degree if you want to get the most out of your Reiki experience, and that it is unwise to take both Degrees back-to-back over a weekend.

We would not take an advanced driving test the day after passing our basic driving test, so why would we believe that moving on to a more 'advanced' level with Reiki would be an effective way to learn when we have had no opportunity to get the hang of the basics of First Degree?

Can we get the most out of Second Degree when we have had no opportunity to get used to working with and sensing and experiencing energy, when we have had no opportunity to enhance our effectiveness as a channel and our sensitivity to Reiki through regular practice, when we have had no opportunity to become familiar with a standard treatment routine and have had no opportunity to feel comfortable and confident in treating other people?

No.

Reiki is not a race, and we need to be familiar with the basics before moving on.

Second Degree is all about:

1. reinforcing or enhancing your connection to the energy
2. learning some symbols which you can use routinely when working on yourself or treating others
3. enhancing your self-healing
4. learning how to effect a strong distant connection (distant healing)

And ideally it is also about opening yourself up to your intuitive side so that you throw away the basic Reiki 'rule book' and go freestyle, gearing any treatments towards the individual needs of the recipient.

There are many approaches to doing these things, and I wanted below to touch on each one and to dispel some myths that may have been passed on.

Enhancing your Connection to the energy

On your Second Degree course you will have received some attunements or some empowerments.
Attunements are not standard rituals within the world of Reiki and take many forms, some simpler and some more complex. They have evolved and changed greatly during their journey from teacher to teacher in the West.

There is no "right way" to carry out an attunement and the individual details of a ritual do not matter a great deal. They all work. Equally, there is no "correct" number of attunements that have to be carried out at

Second Degree level. Whether you receive one, two, or three attunements on your course, that is fine.

On your course you may have received some "empowerments" rather than attunements, though these are less common. The word "empowerment", or "Reiju empowerment", refers to a connection ritual that has come to us from some Japanese sources, and is closer in essence to the empowerment that Mikao Usui conveyed to his students.

If you are receiving empowerments rather than attunements then you really need to have received three of them at least.

What we experience when receiving an attunement or an empowerment will vary a lot. Some people have fireworks and bells and whistles and that's nice for them; other people notice a lot less, or very little, or even nothing, and that's fine too. What we feel when we have an attunement is not a guide to how well it has worked for us. Attunements work, and sometimes we will have a strong experience, but it's not compulsory!

Whether we have noticed a lot, or very little, the attunement will have given us what we need.

Since in Mikao Usui's system you would have received empowerments from him again and again, it would be nice if you could echo this practice by receiving further empowerments (or attunements) and perhaps these might be available at your teacher's Reiki shares or get-togethers, if they hold them.

But it is possible to receive distant Reiju empowerments and various teachers make them freely available as a regular 'broadcast'.

This is not essential, and your connection to Reiki once given does not fizzle out, but it would be a beneficial practice if you could receive regular empowerments from someone.

Being "attuned" to a symbol

For many years within the world of Reiki, people believed that the symbols would not work for you, that they were essentially useless, until you had been "attuned" to the symbol: then it would work for you.

Unfortunately the only connection rituals available in the West were 'attunements' which involved attuning you to a symbol, so no-one knew how to carry out a 'symbol-free' attunement to see if you really needed to be attuned to a symbol for it to work for you.

But in 1999, from Japan, emerged Reiju empowerments, a representation of the empowerments that Usui conferred, and these empowerments do not use symbols. Finally we were able to see if you really needed to be attuned to a symbol for it to work for you.

Lo and behold we discovered that the symbols work fine for people who are connected to the energy using Reiju; they work fine for people who are connected to Reiki but who have not been 'attuned' to the symbols. It seems that once you are connected to Reiki – and now we know how to achieve this without symbols entering into the process – the symbols will work for you, and in fact any symbol seems to push the energy in a particular direction without you having to be specifically 'attuned' to it (whatever that means).

The Reiki symbols are simply graphical representations of different aspects of the energy, a way of representing and emphasising what is already there.

"Sacred Symbols"

In some lineages students are not allowed to keep copies of the symbols and have to reproduce them from memory, based on what they learned on their Second Degree course.

There is the suggestion that the symbols are sacred and not only sacred but secret, and should not be shown to people who are not involved in Reiki, or people who are at First Degree level.

Where this idea came from in the Western Reiki system is not clear, since certainly Dr Hayashi had his students copy out his notes by way of preparing their own manuals, including copying down the symbols.

For me, the Reiki symbols are simply graphical representations of different aspects of the energy, useful tools to assist us in experiencing or becoming consciously aware of different aspects of what we already have, and what is special or sacred is our connection to the source, not the squiggles we might put on a piece of paper.

Because of the 'Chinese whispers' that have resulted from students not being allowed to take home hard copies of the Reiki symbols, there are many different versions of the symbols in existence, but they are mainly variations on a theme and they all seem to work in practice.

Do remember, though, that the original CKR had an anticlockwise spiral, and to use a version of CKR with a clockwise spiral is to use a symbol that is not part of the Usui/Hayashi/Takata system.

Using Symbols in practice

Some students are taught there is one 'correct' way that symbols have to be used. Reiki is not so finicky. The important thing when using a Reiki symbol is to focus your attention on the symbol in some way, so whether you are drawing the symbol with your fingers hovering over the back of your hand as you treat someone, whether you are drawing out the symbol using eye movements, or nose movements, or in your mind's eye, all approaches will work.

You do not need to visualise the symbols in a particular colour and if you can see the symbol in your mind's eye in its entirety – this takes practice - you can 'flash' the whole symbol rather than drawing it out stroke by stroke.

Just because we have been taught some symbols does not mean that we are now obliged to use them all the time when we treat or when we work on ourselves. They can be used to emphasise different aspects of the energy, but this is optional.

Use of symbols does seem to boost the flow of energy, so we can use them when it feels appropriate.

This is the key: to bring a symbol into a particular part of a treatment when we have a strong feeling that we ought to, to work intuitively rather than following a set method.

I have written in other articles about the issue of simplicity within Reiki practice, and the complicated way that people have ended up using the Reiki symbols, for example mixing symbols together or using complicated symbol sandwiches. Remember that the simple approach is usually the most effective, and that there is no hard and fast way that you 'have' to work with the symbols you have been shown.

By the way, if you have been taught that you have to draw the three Second Degree symbols over your palm each day or else they will stop working for you, you can safely ignore these instructions. The symbols will work for you no matter what you do or don't do with your palms!

Why the symbols are there

At Second Degree, the prime focus of Reiki is still your self-healing, and the first two symbols are there to help you get to grips with two important energies that will further or deepen your self-healing.

Putting the 'distant healing' symbol to one side, the other two symbols represent the energies of earth ki and heavenly ki, and we need to fully assimilate these two energies to enhance our self-healing and self-development. If we are going to use these energies when we treat other people, it makes sense to be thoroughly familiar with these energies, to have spent time 'becoming' these energies.

We can do this by carrying out regular symbol meditations.

Making 'distant' connections

The third Reiki symbol that you are introduced to on a Second Degree course is commonly called the 'distant healing symbol'.

We should remember that distant healing is perfectly possible at First Degree level and that we do not need to use a symbol in order to send Reiki to another person: intent is enough. But using this symbol can help us to learn to better 'click' into a nice strong merged state.

There is no set form of ritual that 'has' to be used in distant healing, there is not set form of words that has to be recited, no established sequence which needs to be reproduced in order for distant healing to be effective, so we can find our own comfortable approach, different from other people's but equally valid.

The details of the ritual that we use are not important.

All we need to do is to focus our attention on the recipient and maybe use the symbol in some way, merge with the energy, merge with the recipient, and allow the energy to flow.

Intuitive working

Ideally, Second Degree should be the stage where you start to leave the basic 'rulebook' behind and go 'freestyle', gearing your treatment towards the recipient's individual energy needs, so that each treatment will be different, as the recipient's energy needs change from one treatment session to another.

Some students will already be modifying the basic treatment routine by the time that they arrive on their Second Degree course.

Set hand positions and a prescribed scheme to follow are useful things to have at First Degree, and allow the student to feel confident in treating others, but sequences of hand positions can be left behind when we open to intuition.

Intuitive treatments seem to do something special for the recipient: when you direct the energy into just the right combination of positions for that person on that occasion you allow the energy to penetrate deeply and this seems to lead to a more profound experience for the recipient.

Treatments using intuitively guided hand positions may involve much fewer hand positions being held, and each combination being held for much longer, than in a 'standard' treatment.

We recommend that the Japanese "Reiji ho" approach is used to help Second Degree students to open to their intuitive side, since the approach is so simple and seems to work for most people even within a few minutes of practice. The resulting strong belief that the student is "intuitive" is a hugely empowering state and opens many doors.

Finally

Reiki has the potential to make an amazing, positive difference to you and the people around you.

Remember that Reiki is simplicity itself, and by taking some steps to work on yourself regularly, and share Reiki with the people close to you, you are embarking on a very special journey.

How far you travel on that journey is governed by how many steps you take. Carry on with your Hatsurei and self-treatments, get to grips with the energies of CKR and SHK through regular meditation, find your own comfortable approach to carrying out distant healing, and open yourself to intuitive working.

And have fun!

Course Schedule: Second Degree

Here you can see a basic structure for your Reiki First Degree course, showing what to cover in the morning and afternoon session.

The course is held on a single day and assumes that the student has spent some time before the course reading the course manual and listening to the course audio CDs.

That way, they know a lot about what they are going to be doing on the course and, rather then spending a lot of time as a teacher sitting telling them stuff that they could have read about beforehand, you can concentrate on the practical stuff: helping them to work with energy for their own benefit and to help other people.

So the course is all about summarising and recapping things that the student is already familiar, and putting everything into practice.

Students arrive at 9.30am, starting the course at 10am the latest. Break for lunch, say 45 minutes. Afternoon session starts by 2pm. Finish 5pm – 5.30pm latest

Introduction

See what has happened to the student since Reiki1:
What differences have they noticed within themselves?
How did they get on with establishing a regular routine
of carrying out hatsurei and the self-treatment
meditation? What have they noticed when working on
other people? What feedback have they received?

Remind them of the practices of the original system at
Second Degree

Reiju empowerment # 1: uses focus kotodama

Talk about the use of two symbols to represent earth ki
and heavenly ki and the reasons why we need to get to
grips with these two energies: for personal growth/self-
healing.: experiencing things as they really are.
Meditating on these energies regularly is a powerful self-
healing practice and should replace the self-treatment
meditation regularly.

Meditate on the energy of CKR, and obtain feedback on experiences

Reiju empowerment # 2: uses harmony kotodama

Talk about using these energies when you treat
someone, and how this can be done. Simplest method
is to keep symbol up in the air above you
(recommended), though you can draw/visualise the

symbol over your hands if you like. How to decide which symbol to use.

Meditate on the energy of SHK, compare with CKR, and then back to SHK

Channel CKR energy and SHK energy into each other's temples, & compare

Reiju empowerment # 3: uses connection kotodama

Talk about the importance of Oneness in the original system, how this is a further experience of 'how things really are', and how this has morphed into the idea of distant healing in the Hayashi/Takata system. Talk about different approaches that you can take – some very simple, some more complex - and some of the creative things you can do with DH.

Talk them through a distant healing session for 5 minutes, say. Obtain feedback

[LUNCH]

Talk about the importance of Intent:

Many hands visualisation, energy going where your attention is directed: the important thing is your intent, not what or whether you can visualise. Mention beaming Reiki, radiating Reiki, sending Reiki with your 'eyes' or 'breath'

Practise many hands visualisation on knee/leg

Practise sending 'with eyes' to another's forehead

Perhaps doing distant healing to forehead using intent only (eyes closed)

Talk about working intuitively: introduce 'Reiji ho'

Ideal way to work: benefits for recipient because the treatment is powerful. Benefit for giver since you enter a lovely merged state. Talk about the need to not try, the need to just 'be' with the energy, merge with the energy, no expectations. Mention a ritual you can use.

Take turns on treatment table and practice Reiji ho, moving to different areas of the body every once in a while

Conclude by talking about the importance of working on self regularly, and the simplicity of the original system, the importance of intent/intuition, and letting the energy guide you

Suggested points to make on the Second Degree course

These are some notes, based on the sort of points that I make on my courses, for information and guidance. I do not expect you to say the same things as me, and I do not expect you to only make these points, but the following notes give you an idea of some of the things that could be said

The important thing is to keep things simple, remind students of the basic practices of the original system as they progress through the course, and to emphasise personal responsibility: they need to go away and do the work regularly to obtain the benefits that are available through Reiki.

Morning session

Your Introduction

It is nice by way of introduction to get the students to talk about what has been happening since their Reiki1 course. They could mention four areas:

1. Whether they have felt any changes within themselves since learning Reiki
2. How did they get on with establishing a routine of working on themselves using hatsurei and the self-treatment meditation?
3. What have they noticed when treating other people?
4. What feedback have they received from the people they have worked on?

I introduce them to the course, summarise what is going to happen during the day, and explain why I have sent the manuals out in advance: much better to spend time on the course doing things with energy rather than practising drawing symbols.

They have been 'mollycoddled'! Most people don't get to see the symbols until the day of the course and then have to learn them under pressure on the day. They have had ages to learn them, so no excuses!!

Reminder of the original system at Second Degree

The original system, even at Second Degree, was not focused on the treatment of others, though some treatments might have been carried out at this level, and if they were, the approach was simple and intuitive.

The system continued the basic focus of First Degree, with the students living the precepts and practising mindfulness, with regular Reiju empowerments being received, and with a basic practice of energy work.

What we do at Second Degree is to introduce two important energies for the student to work with: the energies of earth ki and heavenly ki, and meditating on these energies regularly is an important self-healing practice that can be substituted for the self-treatment meditation on a regular basis.

Students were also introduced to the experience of a state of oneness, and this has morphed into the practice of distant healing in the Hayashi/Takata system used on most Reiki courses.

Our courses are trying to get to back to the focus of the original practice, while still including a treatment emphasis (so that these courses are reasonably compatible with the general run of Western-style Reiki courses), and presenting the original practices in a way that will work for a modern Western audience.

The precepts were the very foundation of the system, and as much development was said to be possible through following the precepts as would come through carrying out the energy work.

At Second Degree we can continue to work with the precepts and learn to live our lives in accordance with them, through considering them in turn and deciding for ourselves how they impinge on your behaviour, reactions and relationships.

It would be useful if the student spent some time reading about mindfulness and trying to make this a part of their life.

We provide Reiju empowerments in person on this course, and then at a distance each week on Mondays, for students to tune into.

The course will equip the student to carry out the new symbol-based energy exercises, with an audio CD to talk the student through the exercises.

And we cover the treatment of others fully, so that the course is compatible with the 'treatment' focus of most Reiki courses.

Giving the First Empowerment: uses the focus kotodama

I tell them that I am not going to suggest to them what they might notice when receiving an empowerment, because I don't want to put ideas into their head. I tell them that they will be sitting quietly with their hands resting in their laps, listening to the music and feeling themselves becoming peaceful and relaxed.

When it is their turn to receive their empowerment I will rest my hand on their shoulder, which is a cue for them to bring their hands into the prayer position. I will carry out their empowerment, which does not involve touching them or making contact with them, and when the empowerment is over I'll bring their hands back down into their lap.

Then they will wait quietly with their eyes closed until I have finished with everyone else, and then I'll bring them all back together.

… and then we'll see what they noticed, not because I'm looking for a particular thing, but because it's nice to see how experiences vary from one person to another.

I remind the students that what they feel when they receive an empowerment is no guide to how well it has worked.

People's experiences vary greatly from one person to another. Some people seem to naturally notice a lot more happening than others.

Introducing them to symbols

We need to understand why the symbols are there. The original system was all about working on yourself to develop spiritually and to enhance self-healing.

At Second Degree the student moved on from the basic practices of First Degree to work with two powerful energies, two powerful aspects of their being, because doing so enhances self-healing and spiritual development.

A lot of the students chanted Shinto mantras or used special meditations to get two grips with the energies of earth ki and heavenly ki, but symbols can be used for this purpose too.

Meditating on these energies regularly is a powerful self-healing practice.

The idea behind the use of these energies is that earth ki and heavenly ki are two aspects of our being – our physical reality and our spiritual essence.

The idea is that what we are is physical reality and spiritual essence, and by coming to experience fully our physical reality and our spiritual essence we are being led to experience things as they really are – one of the goals of Buddhism in fact – and to do so is a powerful tool for self-healing.

CKR energy

Tell them how they can carry out a meditation to experience earth ki. They put the symbol up in the air above them and say its name to themselves silently three times.

They then draw down energy from CKR above, down to their Tanden, and spread the energy through their body and beyond, and see how that feels.

Obtain feedback from all the students, and explain how you feel the energies.

I then get the students to tell me the names of CKR and SHK, and get them to say out loud the names three times, in a jokey way.

It helps to make them comfortable with the pronunciation to hear me and the other students saying the names out loud. At intervals I get them to remind me of the names of CKR and SHK!

Giving the Second Empowerment: uses the harmony kotodama

Tell them that the first empowerment they had flooded them with earth ki, and that the second empowerment will flood them with heavenly ki... so two different flavours.

SHK meditation

We do a meditation where they draw down energy from SHK above them and see how that feels for a while, then they scrub out that symbol and replace it with CKR and experience that energy for a while, finally scrubbing out CKR and going back to drawing down energy from SHK again for a while.

How did the SHK energy feel, and how did it compare with that of CKR? What is the difference between the two?

Explain how you feel the two energies.

Using symbols to treat people

Here are the general points that I make on the course, recapping on what they have already read in the manual and listened to on the audio CD:

- You can use the energies of earth ki and heavenly ki when you treat someone. Using a symbol boosts the flow of energy and pushes the energy in a particular direction, making treatments more intense.
- Because you have learned the Reiki symbols does not mean that you are now obliged to use them all the time. You can still do 'Reiki1 treatments' where you let the energy flow, and you can see these treatments more as gentle introductory treatments. Sometimes it may feel right to ease the person into the energy gently. But by using the symbols you make the treatment more intense.
- Whenever you use any of the Reiki symbols you will always be drawing or visualising the symbol once and saying the symbol's name silently to yourself three times. It's the combination of drawing it out and saying its name that produces its effect
- The easiest way to use a symbol when you treat is to put it up in the air above you and say its name three times (as in the meditation). Energy flows down to you as you treat, down to your

Tanden; energy flows out of your hands. This is the way we recommend

- You can draw the symbol out in different ways, though. You can draw great big flamboyant symbols on the wall of a treatment room, using the palm of your hand. You can bunch your fingers together and draw a symbol over the back of your hand as you treat. If your hands are 'otherwise engaged' you can use nose/head movements or eye movements to tract out a symbol over your hands. You can draw the symbol in your mind's eye above you, and imagine energy cascading down to you from above. There is no one way of drawing the symbol.
- The first two symbols are used routinely when treating people. They produce two quite distinctive energies.

So CKR produces a low frequency energy that can be seen as focusing on the physical body. You can see it as a physical healing energy.

Usui's surviving students see this energy as earth ki, the energy of physical reality, physical existence. You can use this energy anywhere you like in the body. It boosts the flow of energy and focuses the energy on physical healing.

SHK produces a higher frequency energy that focuses on thoughts and emotions, producing mental balance, emotional release. Usui's surviving students see this energy as heavenly ki, connecting you with your spiritual essence. In practice this symbol would be used over the head and solar plexus, the main areas of mental and emotional activity, though if you have a strong feeling that it should be used in a particular area then just go with that.

Using CKR and SHK energies on each other

The students then spend some time sending these two energies into each other. One person sits in a chair and the other stands behind. The person standing up then visualises CKR up in the air above them – saying the name three times of course – and draws energy down from the symbol into their crown, and sends the energy out of their hands into the temples of the recipient.

After a while they replace the symbol with SHK and carry on sending energy into the recipient's temples.

After a while you get feedback from the recipients. I tell them that they should be read to give adjectives to describe what they felt. If they felt heat, what sort of heat was it? Was it gentle or coarse, fierce, superficial or deeply penetrating. How did the energy feel? What impressions did they have of it?

Sometimes the sender will have felt a difference too, and they should be asked about that, but a greater difference is usually noticed by the recipient.

Then the students swap over and repeat the exercise, so they have all been on the receiving end and sent the energy too.

Giving the Third Empowerment: uses the connection kotodama

Tell them that the final empowerment they will receive will flood them with the essence of the distant healing symbol. They will experience a state of oneness.

Carrying on the theme of 'experiencing things as they really are', the ultimate reality is that of oneness: moving into a state where there is no me, there is no you. We move beyond the 'illusion' of our existence to experience true reality from the Buddhist perspective: that of oneness.

Again, most of Usui's students chanted Shinto mantras or used special meditations in order to experience a state of oneness, but we can use symbols to achieve the same thing, and there is a symbol used in Reiki which has become referred to as the distant healing symbol.

Distance healing is an expression of oneness (treating someone is also an expression of oneness, actually).

Usui's students wouldn't have carried out distant healing as we understand it, though they would have realised that they could do this easily. They would have believed that by working on themselves they were also working on other people.

What we can do by way of echoing the original practice is to carry out distant healing to give us the experience of oneness, and that will benefit us as much as the receiver: when we carry out distant healing we also heal ourselves.

Distant healing

This is what I tell them about distant healing, recapping on what they have already read in the manual and heard on the audio CD...

There are no hard and fast rules when it comes to distant healing. The bare bones are to know where you want to send the energy – you set a definite intent – and you use the distant healing symbol in some way to access that distant connection.

Beyond that, the details of what ritual you use are up to you. Some people like to set up quite a detailed and complicated ritual, and that's fine, but a simple approach works just as well.

In fact you do not even need to use a symbol to carry out distant healing, though the symbol does act as a trigger that helps you to click more into a state of oneness, and using the symbol can help you to better recognise and more easily move into that state.

The simplest approach would then be to focus your attention on the recipient, feel yourself merging with the energy and the recipient, and just be empty and still, no expectations.

An alternative would be to carry out the 'self-treatment meditation' but instead of imagining that you are treating a carbon copy of yourself, you could imagine that you are treating the recipient, sitting on the floor in front of you.

Some people use a prop, like a teddy bear or a doll. They draw the distant symbol over the doll and Reiki the doll with the intention that the energy is being sent to the recipient. Some people use their leg to represent the person.

A technique that I like is to run through some memories of a person, or imagine them in their usual surroundings, to make a strong connection to them. Then imagine that they are being shrunk down so that they fit in the palm

247

of your hand... so you have made a strong connection with them and brought their essence to your palm.

Then you draw the distant symbol over your palm, say the name three times, and cup one hand over the other, sending Reiki through an 'energy tube' passing from your hands to the recipient. Then you can actively visualise, seeing the recipient engulfed with healing energy, or see yourself carrying out a treatment on them, or you can keep it really simple and feel yourself blending or merging with the energy.

In practice distant healing tends to be carried out for 10-15 minutes at a time over a number of consecutive days: say, 3-5 days.

If you send distant Reiki to someone and they do not know it is coming: maybe they are shopping at the supermarket, then they probably won't notice anything having happened. That's not to say they didn't receive the energy, it just means that they weren't consciously aware of having received it.

To obtain feedback from the recipient you'll need to set a particular time – to make an appointment with them – for them to sit down at the allotted time in a quiet room without too many distractions, close their eyes, and see what happens.

If you want to send Reiki to lots of people, you could find yourself sitting up all night if you take 15 minutes for each person, so it is possible to send Reiki to many people at the same time by using a distant healing book or a distant healing box.

You write the recipients' names in the book, or have them on pieces of paper in the box, you review the list of names, draw the distant healing symbol over the box/book, and then Reiki the book/box with the intention that the energy is being sent to all the recipients.

You can send Reiki to deal with events or situations that have had a long-term effect in terms of the way that you think or feel about things. Visualise the situation or event, draw the distant healing symbol over the situation, and send Reiki to the situation to heal the ripples, to heal the effects that this event has produced within you.

You can send Reiki to the future, with the intention that it is going to be received at a particular time, or conditional on something happening. So people have sent Reiki to a public speaking engagement or a job interview, to be received, for example, "when I walk into the interview room".

To gain confidence with distant healing you need to set up some guinea pigs who are going to sit down every evening to receive Reiki and give you feedback. Then you can play around with it.

Say that you have arranged for someone to sit down for 10 minutes every evening, Monday to Friday. Well, don't send anything on Monday, send in real time on Tuesday, on Wednesday send Reiki out at lunchtime with the intention that it is going to be received at the time you specify, and so on. See what response you get.

Distant healing practice

Then I talk the students through a distant healing session lasting for 5 minutes or so, and ask for feedback on what they experienced. Quite often they will have really felt a strong connection with the recipient, or felt that they were there with them, or that they had just 'gone' or merged with the energy; a lovely state to be in.

I point out that with practice it becomes easier and easier to click into that lovely merged state.

Afternoon session

The importance of intent

This part of the course is about showing that the energy is controlled by our intent, effortlessly, that where we focus our attention is where the energy goes. Visualisation is a good method to use to focus our intent, but whether we can visualise something or not, it is the underlying intent that is the important thing, not our ability to visualise.

We can carry out a number of exercises to demonstrate how much effortless control we have over the flow of energy...

The 'Many hands' technique

The students practise this on each other. One person is on the treatment table, and the other rests their hands on the nearest knee, one hand on the other.

They let the energy flow for a while and notice what is going on in their hands, as a baseline to compare things with.

Then they bring in the extra sets of arms and hands, with the hands resting on the ankle, on the upper leg, and in other treatment positions. They imagine that Reiki is flooding down all the sets of arms and out of all the set of hands, into the various treatment positions.

What usually happens is that to begin with the recipient can feel energy quite well localised to the knee. When the extra hands are introduced the energy seems to spread out, being felt over a wider area.

Sometime the recipient can feel discrete 'hands' on their leg, which tie in with the positions of the imaginary hands. Sometimes the recipient can even tell which imaginary hand is put down first!

I explain that the energy follows your thoughts, follows your focus, so if you let your attention dwell in a number of positions at the same time, the energy flows there.

So when you carry out a standard treatment you could treat both sides of the body at the same time, by having some hands 'mirroring' your own. You could be treating the temples and bring imaginary hands behind and in front of the head.

Visualising something is a good way of focusing your intent in a particular way, but what's important is the underlying intent.

Sending with the eyes

This exercise (described in a later section of this guide) can also be used as a good demonstration of the many ways that we can send energy, just by thinking about it.

Sending with the eyes and the breath

From Japan come a couple of techniques where you send Reiki 'with your eyes' or 'with your breath'. I do not think that Reiki is really coming out of your eyes or your mouth.

You are just constructing a ritual that focuses the energy in a particular way, so if you send Reiki 'with your breath' then it picks up on some of the connotations of breathing and is received in a superficial, 'billowing' form which moves quickly from where it was sent to where it was needed.

Reiki sent 'with the eyes' is received in much more of a focused way, it is well localised, piercing, penetrating… picking up on the connotations of staring and focusing. Basically you are sending the energy to the other person, and because of what you imagine that you are doing, the energy picks up on that.

Reinforce how simple it all is: you intend that the energy passes in a particular way and it does. Reiki has few limitations. It is there with you all the time, following your thoughts, following your focus.

Send Reiki to the forehead via distant healing, using intent

This exercise takes things further, and shows that we do not even need to use the imagined intermediary of the eyes in order to send a blast of Reiki to someone's forehead. Focus your attention somewhere and the energy will go there.

Working with Intuition: Reiji ho

This forms the biggest chunk of the afternoon session, and the students will be practising Reiji ho on each other, taking turns to be on the treatment table, so everyone gets the chance to practise on a few different people.

I start by telling the students that they are already intuitive, that they already know exactly the right positions to put their hands on each person they treat, but their conscious minds sit there like a great big lump, preventing them from getting access to the intuitive information that is already there.

I tell them that Usui's way of working was intuitive, that there were no set hand positions and that you allowed the energy to guide you. In practice, using intuitively-guided hand positions leads to treatments that are deeper, more relevant, more profound for the recipients, and it is a lovely way to work because of the deep 'merged' state that you get yourself into in order to access intuitive working.

Reiji ho isn't really a technique, it is just a way of distracting your conscious mind, a way of getting your mind out of the way to allow the intuitive information to come through.

This technique will only work when you don't try, when you don't force it, it will only work when you are in neutral, merged with the energy, and letting it happen in a neutral way.

In practice what you are going to be doing is to hover your hands in a loose, neutral, comfortable position over the person.

You don't make any deliberate hand-movements. You merge with the energy and allow your hands to drift. You become aware of any gentle or subtle pull on your hands, and you allow your hands to drift, rather like being pulled by invisible magnets to the right place to treat.

Sometimes when you do this, your hands will drift and stop in the same position, so no matter where you are by the recipient, your hands come to rest in the same position; there is one 'priority area' for the recipient.

Sometimes, depending on where you are standing by the treatment table, you might be guided to some different positions, so there are a number of priority areas for that person.

Occasionally you might find that your hands keep moving, along a section of a meridian perhaps, or following a strange repeated circuit which carries on for a while before moving on elsewhere.

Sometimes your hands can drift away from the body, sometimes embarrassingly far away from the body! Just allow the energy to guide you.

When your hands come to rest you will usually find that there is a lot going on in your hands, because you have just been guided to an area that was drawing lots of energy.

You stay there until the flow of energy subsides and then let your hands move on to the next combination of positions.

When I treat I start by treating the shoulders, because it gets the energy flowing, and makes them all calm and serene. I then let the energy guide me when I treat the head – and I usually end up with non-symmetrical hand positions (e.g. one side of the throat and one side of the crown, side of the head and front of the face). Then I move on to the torso and let the energy guide me there.

A few practical points are these:

1. Sometimes one hand won't move, because you've hovered it in quite a good position already, just by chance.
2. If your hands are drawn towards the body, do open your eyes to see what part of the body you're just about to touch.
3. When you hover your hands, do have in mind the 'contours' of the person in front of you to make sure your hands don't bash into a part of the body you really ought not to touch.

When this method was first taught in the West, a particular ritual was suggested. Now like most Reiki rituals, the details are optional and you don't have to follow this in practice, but this is what was suggested:

- Put your hands in the prayer position and close your eyes; remind yourself that you have a strong connection to the source.
- Move your hands up so they rest against your forehead (third eye), so you are making a ritual connection between your hands and your intuitive centre.
- With your hands still resting against your third eye, say silently to yourself/to the universe "Please let me be guided", "Please let my hands be guided", "Show me where to treat".

- Slowly move your hands down so that they are hovering in a loose comfortable position over the person.

Now you need to distract yourself, so start to focus your attention on the source, on the energy that is flooding down into your crown.

As the energy flows through your arms and hands, feel yourself disappearing into the energy, imagine yourself becoming one with the energy, merging with it. Just be still, be there with the energy, merge with the energy... and allow your hands to drift.

I have one person on the treatment table and the others arranged around the table (not at the head or the foot of the table because there is less room for the hands to drift: you get more spectacular drifting when you are practising by a long part of the body).

After a while, the students will move round the table so they can practise in the position that another student has stood in, to see if their hands drift into the same sort of positions.

This is reassuring for them, and helps them to believe that they are not just 'making it up'. It is also reassuring if they find that their hands have 'clunked' into another person's hands, as they have both been guide (with their eyes closed) to the same area of the body.

It is doubly reassuring if the hand positions tie in with a particular problem that the recipient has, though this will not always happen.

I encourage and reassure the students as soon as they start to experience their hands drifting, and point out that this method gets easier and easier to do with practice.

Like many of the original Reiki techniques, they are fairly easy to do, they work to an extent the first time you use them, but they get a lot more effective with practice... so while their hands might move quite slowly to begin with, with practice their hands will drift more quickly, more consistently and definitely.

So regular practice is important.

Each time they treat someone they should practise getting into that lovely merged state of mind, and it will become easier and easier to work intuitively. Over time they will also start to attract other intuitive information.

Conclusion to the day

Just like First Degree, Second Degree is focused on the self. The student should be in the routine of carrying out hatsurei and the self-treatment meditation regularly, and now we can move things on my carrying out symbol meditations (CKR and SHK) instead of the self-treatment meditation some of the time.

We can also carry out some distant healing in order to start to experience a state of oneness, and to heal ourselves.

Students should be thinking about the precepts, maybe experimenting with mindfulness, tuning into weekly Reiju empowerments, and these continue at this level.

When treating others, Second Degree gives us some tools to use to make treatments more intense, by focusing on earth ki or heavenly ki when we treat, and by working intuitively.

Reiki 2 Practical Exercises

The Reiki2 exercises revolve around becoming familiar with the energies of CKR and SHK mainly.

Meditating on the energy of CKR and SHK

Here is a way of experiencing the energies of the symbols through meditation, and this should be carried out for 3-5 minutes for each symbol.

1. Sit comfortably with your eyes closed, with your hands resting in your lap and your palms facing upwards.
2. Visualise, say, CKR up in the air above you and say the symbol's name three times silently to yourself to 'empower' the symbol.
3. As you breathe in, draw energy down from the symbol. The energy passes through your crown, down the centre of your body to your Tanden.
4. As you pause before exhaling, feel the energy getting stronger in your Tanden.
5. As you exhale, flood the energy of CKR throughout your body.

261

You will have noticed that this exercise is a variation on Joshin Kokkyu Ho, but we have added the focus on a Reiki symbol.

The symbol, imagined up in the air above you, represents the source of the energy, and doing this is a way of saying to yourself 'I just want the energy of earth ki to flow through me'.

You visualise the symbol at the beginning of the exercise and you do not need to keep the symbol clear in your mind's eye for every second of the meditation.

Visualising with a definite intent at the commencement of the exercise is sufficient, though you may choose to 'renew' the symbol by drawing it out again and saying its name to yourself three times again, at some stage during the meditation.

But do not go overboard with repeating the symbol as you meditate: this is unnecessary.

How do you feel? What sensations or impressions are you getting?

How does the energy affect you in terms of your physical sensations and impressions, your mental state, your mental activity, your emotions?

Use earth ki or heavenly ki when you treat someone

One person sits in a chair with their eyes closed and gets ready to describe what they experience.

Another person stands behind them and gets ready with to channel energy into the recipient's temples. What they do is this:

In their mind's eye they will draw out a great big CKR up in the air above them, say its name three times, and imagine cascades of energy flooding down to them from the symbol above them, flooding down to their Tanden.

The energy then flows out of their hands into the person in front of them. All the time more and more energy floods down to them from the symbol above them.

Do this exercise for a few minutes.

To bring the exercise to an end, they imagine the symbol disintegrating and disappearing, and feel the flow of energy subside.

Then in their mind's eye they will draw out a great big SHK up in the air above them, say its name three times, and imagine cascades of energy flooding down to them from the symbol above them, flooding down to their Tanden.

263

The energy then flows out of their hands into the person in front of them. All the time more and more energy floods down to them from the symbol above them. Do this exercise for a few minutes.

To bring the exercise to an end, they imagine the symbol disintegrating and disappearing, and feel the flow of energy subside.

Obtain feedback from the recipient: how did the two energies feel, what did they experience? Obtain feedback from the sender: how did they perceive the energy?

Send Reiki with the eyes

This is a good exercise to carry out to demonstrate the importance of intent. I don't believe that Reiki does actually come out of the eyes, like Clark Kent (Superman in disguise) sending laser beams out of his eyes. I believe that we are simply intending that the energy passes to the other person, and the 'eye technique' is simply a little 'construct', a ritual that focuses our intent in a particular way.

But the energy seems to pick up on some of the connotations of staring and breathing, so Reiki sent with the breath seems to be received in a billowing, superficial way, whereas Reiki sent with the eyes seems to be received in more of a piercing, penetrating, focused way.

Arjava Petter says that the key to directing Reiki with the eyes seems to be to defocus the eyes, to look with soft focus, to look through the area where we want to send the energy, and to intend that the energy travels with your gaze.

He says that you should look 'with a loving state of being' behind you.

This exercise is done in pairs. One person sits in a chair with their eyes closed, and gets ready to describe what they experience. Another person sits opposite them and gets ready to send three 'blasts' of Reiki to the recipient's forehead.

We send to the forehead because we are quite sensitive to the energy there and we are more likely to notice something happening there.

The sender looks away to begin with, to make sure they are not sending Reiki by mistake, and they focus on the floor. When they are ready to send they look at the receiver's forehead and say out loud "Sending".

They send a stream of Reiki to the forehead for 10-15 seconds and then look away again, saying out loud "Looking Away" as they do so.

The sender tells the receiver when they are sending and not sending so that the recipient can tie in their experiences with when the sender says that they are sending – and not sending - the energy.

In my experience, most people will feel something happening when the energy is sent. The energy will be perceived in many different ways though: as colours, as pressure, as heat/fizzing, as white light, as a headache. There are many variations.

This exercise helps students to realise that there are many ways of sending Reiki: with your hands, distantly, through beaming, through intent (eye and breath being a good example of this), radiating it out of your whole body.

Send Reiki to the forehead via distant healing, using intent (optional)

This is a variation on the 'eye' exercise, which demonstrates the power of intent, shows how simple distant healing can be, and shows that you don't need to use your eyes to send energy to someone's forehead!

This exercise is done in pairs. Both sender and receiver sit in a chair with their eyes closed; the receiver gets ready to describe what they experience.

The sender sits near them (they do not need to sit facing the receiver) and gets ready to send three 'streams' of Reiki to the recipient's forehead.

The teacher gives a countdown "three... two... one... send!" and the sender then focuses their attention on the receiver's forehead and allows their attention to dwell there, the energy focusing there.

After about 10-15 seconds the teacher says out loud "stop sending". Then repeat a couple of more times.

Obtain feedback about the sender's and receiver's experiences.

Alternative Course Schedule for Second Degree

Tina Shaw has been experimenting with a different format for Second Degree courses and it seems to be working very well.

She was reacting to some comments from her students who were a bit disappointed that they did not get to do a treatment on each other on the course – only practising exercises rather than using them for real. So what Tina has done is this:

Changes to the morning session

In the morning you do symbol meditations with the students as normal but you don't have them practise using the energies on each other (that comes in the afternoon).

By leaving out the 'using symbols on each other' part of the morning session, this saves a bit of time and there would definitely be time to be able to go through distant healing with students before lunch (I think some of you might do this after lunch sometimes).

Changes to the afternoon session

The afternoon begins with a description of what they are going to be doing, talking about channelling CKR/SHK, 'many hands' and Reiji ho.

Then there is a general "all in" Reiji ho practice session, all practising on each other (one person on the table and the others all practising at the same time) so they can get the feel of what they are going to be doing later in the main part of the afternoon.

Tina feels that it would probably work better (take less time) if the teacher was on the table; I think there is enough time for students to rotate, even with the two treatment sessions that follow (see below).

Then the students get to treat each other, a bit like they did on the Reiki 1 course, but this time they get to put into practice the new techniques that are introduced on Second Degree:

1. Go through the usual Affirm, Connect, Build, Merge, Flow routine from First Degree.
2. Go to shoulders and treat shoulders for a few minutes to get the energy going.
3. Stay at shoulders and spend a few minutes channelling CKR energy
4. Stay at shoulders and spend a few minutes channelling SHK energy
5. Move hands to temples and treat for a couple of minutes and then add sets of extra hands that

hover over the face and (optional) cup round the back of the head. Treat like this for a few minutes

6. Ask student to move to the side of the recipient and place their hands in prayer position, against their third eye, and ask to be guided. Student spends about 20 minutes using Reiji ho, letting the energy guide their hands. If they like they can send some CKR or SHK or do some 'many hands' as they do this; they can decide whether to add these in or not.

7. They finish on the feet for a few minutes and smooth down the energy field at the end as usual.

The creates approx 40 minute treatment from very beginning to very end.

Reiki Master
Teacher course

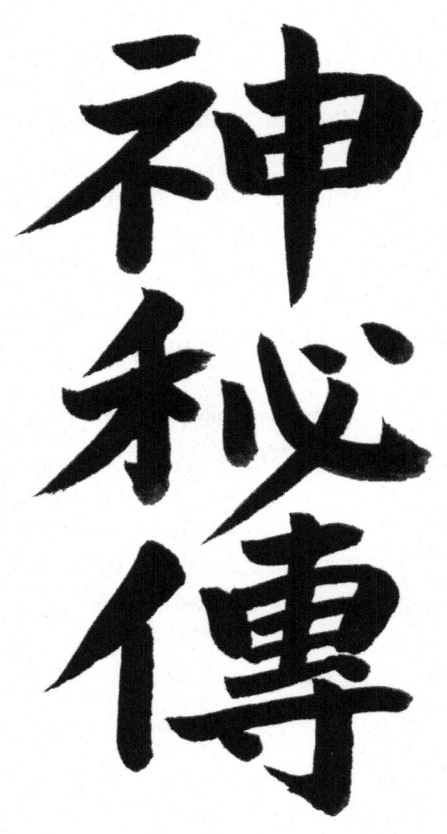

This guide is designed to give you a general outline for the carrying out of my Reiki Master / Teacher course.

You will find a description of the main themes of the course, the course schedule, suggestions for the main points to get across at each stage of the course, and practical exercises to use with the students.

This course is based on 18-20 hours of pre-course study/exercises followed by two full day's training, equivalent to a five-day course.

The two 'live' days are to a large extent a way of:

- recapping on things that the students are already reasonably familiar with
- putting the things they have read about into practice
- clarifying things that may not be completely clear
- focusing on the main 'themes' of the course, putting things into context

The two days of the live course should not be about imparting a lot of new information, since that is the most ineffective and inefficient way of teaching and learning.

I have included a lot of 'accelerated learning' techniques within the course.

The course materials cater for different learning styles, and effective learning comes about more easily if the student has the opportunity to do these things:

1. Read text
2. Listen to things: commentary and instructions
3. Look at images, cartoons, mind maps, summaries
4. Watch live (or video) demonstrations
5. Imagine themselves carrying out tasks
6. Talk out loud to explain things to other students
7. Make physical movements to explain things or in response to other people's instructions

… and students will be doing all these things in different combinations during the pre-course study and live course.

The Course Materials

These materials are sent to the students about 6 weeks before the course:

- Reiki Master / Teacher Course manual
- Two RMT Course Audio CDs, lasting nearly 2 hours
- DVD
- Pre-Course instructions

Pre-Course Activities

Instead of learning about Western attunements for the first time on the day of the course, learning about Reiju empowerments for first time on the day of the course, meditating on the two Master symbols for the first time on the day of the course, and being introduced to the Kotodama, the power of Intent and Intuitive working for the first time on the day of the course… far better for these areas to all be fairly familiar to the students already, so that the course itself can be mainly practical: doing things with energy, clarifying and recapping, putting things into context, concentrating on the main points and themes that need to be understood.

During the pre-course period, the students will be doing these things:

- Familiarising themselves with the contents of the course: the course materials, the subjects to be covered. They will get an overview of the manual, listen to the audio CDs, watch the DVD maybe.
- Reading (and listening) about Reiki symbols and learning some of them: Tibetan DKM, Usui DKM, Fire Dragon, Spirit Column, Mental Spiral, Heart Chakra symbol
- Spend two weeks meditating each day on the energies of the Tibetan DKM and Usui DKM to get to grips with the symbols' energies on the run-up to the live course.
- Reading (and listening) about the Kotodama, Intent and Intuition.
- Learning how to carry out Second Degree attunements.
- Learning how to carry out Reiju empowerments.

By the time the students arrive the live course they will have:

- learned five symbols and will be able to draw them easily for memory, particularly the "Tibetan" Master Symbol and the Usui Master Symbol.

275

- meditated on the energies of the "Tibetan" and Usui Master Symbols each day for a fortnight, and kept some notes on how their energies feel.

- become familiar with the process of Reiju empowerments and know how they can be used at the different Reiki levels.

- become familiar with the Second Degree Reiki attunement method and have practised the "Violet Breath" technique.

Main Themes of the Course

Here is a diagram (below) to show the main themes that are dealt with on this course:

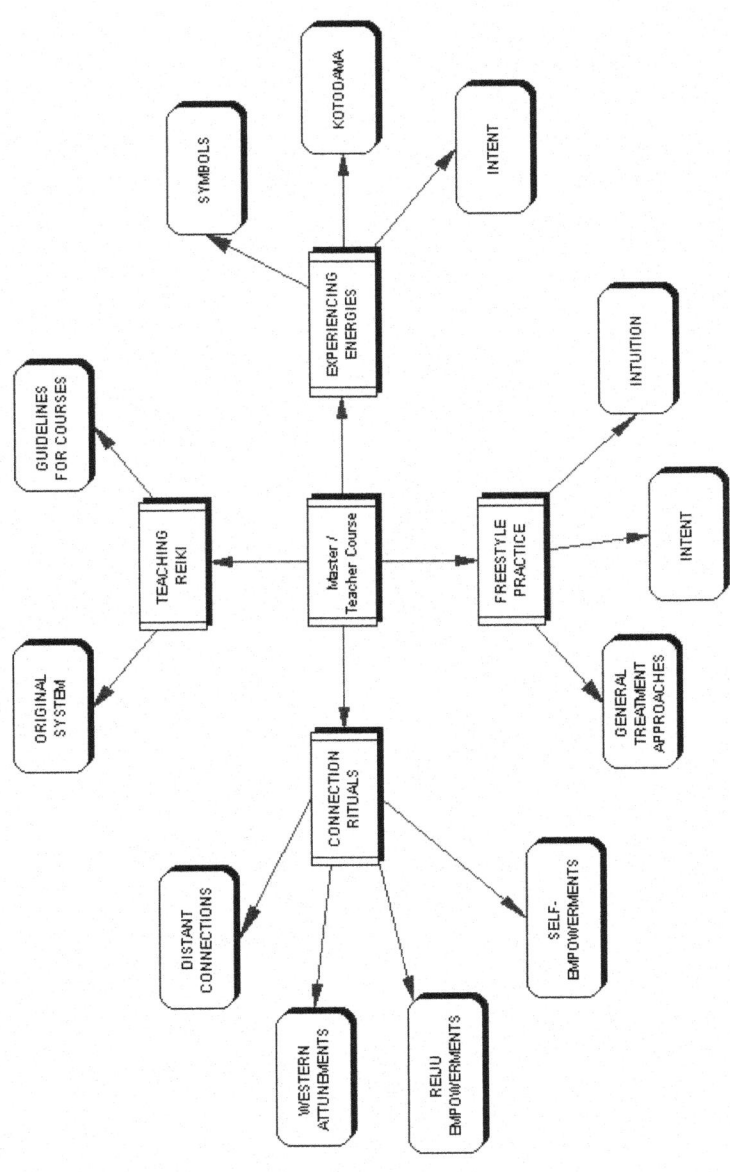

SYMBOLS

KOTODAMA

INTENT

EXPERIENCING ENERGIES

GUIDELINES FOR COURSES

TEACHING REIKI

ORIGINAL SYSTEM

Master / Teacher Course

INTUITION

FREESTYLE PRACTICE

INTENT

GENERAL TREATMENT APPROACHES

CONNECTION RITUALS

DISTANT CONNECTIONS

WESTERN ATTUNEMENTS

REIJU EMPOWERMENTS

SELF-EMPOWERMENTS

277

Afternoon sessions

The two afternoons of the course focus on connections: Western attunements, Reiju empowerments, distant attunements/empowerments and self-empowerments.

The Saturday afternoon deals with Western attunements and the Sunday afternoon deals with Reiju, distant connections and self-empowerments (including experiencing the energy of the empowerment kotodama through chanting).

Morning sessions

The morning sessions deal with Experiencing energies (using symbols, kotodama and intent), treatments, intent and intuition.

So on the Saturday morning they learn about the original system and the role of symbols in Reiki, talking about their experiences of meditating on the two Master symbols, and they experience the energies of the Second Degree kotodama, learning how symbols and kotodama can be used on themselves and others.

On the Sunday morning we get to grips with the power of intent and the potential of intuition, going through various exercises to demonstrate what is possible.

Empowerments & attunements given

The empowerments/attunements that I carry out are as follows:

Sat am   Hatsurei followed by empowerment
                (using empowerment kotodama)

Sat pm   Western Master attunement

Sun am   Kenyoku/Joshin Kokkyu ho followed by
                empowerment (using empt kotodama)

Sun pm   "Plain" Reiju

Getting to grips with the course content

I think that the best way to get to grips with content and main points/themes of this course would be to listen to the two audio CDs first, which last for nearly two hours and cover the main things that I would say on the day of a course, and more.

They give you a broad overview of the content and focus you on the main themes and ideas that we convey to students.

Don't listen to all the tracks all in one go: the best way would be to:

1. Focus on one particular area at a time
2. Look at the relevant section of the Reiki Master Teacher course manual
3. Look at the course schedule
4. Look at the guidelines below
5. Listen to the relevant audio track a few times

Then imagine yourself going through the course, what you would say, what you would hope to achieve etc.

Practise saying things out loud, so you get used to putting things into your own words and become familiar with explaining ideas in a comfortable way.

The tracks of the audio CDs are as follows:

Master / Teacher Audio CD 1

1	Welcome	2.42m
2	The Original System	5.18m
3	Experiencing Energies	2.56m
4	Symbols and Treatments	8.28m
5	The Kotodama	5.26m
6	Intent	7.10m
7	Intuition	4.02m
8	Non-Reiki techniques	10.09m
9	Reiju empowerments	9.37m
10	Western attunements	6.34m
11	Thoughts on Usui System	1.41m
12	Teaching Reiki	5.29m

Master / Teacher Audio CD 2

1	Reiju empowerment instructions	8.20m
2	Reiki2 attunement guide	16.36m
3	Frequency Scale meditation	8.16m
4	Reiji ho instructions	7.40m

Course Schedule

Saturday morning

Overview of the Course
Receive a Reiju empowerment at Master level.
Overview of Usui Sensei's system and how we can echo
the original approaches
Experiencing energies using Symbols: focusing on the
Master Symbols, and the use of Symbols when working
on yourself and others
Experiencing energies using the Reiki Kotodama: find
out how to use them on yourself and others

Saturday afternoon

Overview: Western-style attunements
Receive a 'Western' Master attunement.
Learn how to attune others 'Western' style, using
Second Degree as an example.
Learn how to attune at Master level and First Degree
level.

Sunday morning

Receive a Reiju empowerment at Master level.
Review of Day One: any questions?
The importance of intent: directing energy using
intent/visualisation, and 'frequency setting'

Working with intuition: expanding our experience of Reiji ho, perceiving the chakras, and "mind's eye" visual shortcuts.

Sunday afternoon

Receive a Reiju empowerment.
Learn how to carry our Reiju empowerments and practice on each other.
Learn how Reiju can be use at different levels and practice on each other.
The benefits of Reiju
Distant connections
The empowerment Kotodama
Learn how to empower yourself.
Conclusion

The above schedule assumes that you are running the course over two consecutive days on a weekend.

Some teachers prefer to run the course with a gap of a week in between day 1 and day 2. This can work really well, and gives an opportunity for things learned and recapped on day 1 to really sink in before the student moves on.

Students also have an opportunity to put what they learned into practice and may well have questions and ideas come to them in the intervening period, which they can then follow up with the teacher on day 2.

Saturday morning

1. Overview of the Course
2. Receive a Reiju empowerment at Master level.
3. Overview of Usui Sensei's system and how we can echo the original approaches
4. Experiencing energies using Symbols: focusing on the Master Symbols, and the use of Symbols when working on yourself and others
5. Experiencing energies using the Reiki Kotodama: find out how to use them on yourself and others

Guidelines

Start by giving the students an overview of the main themes of the course, letting them know in general terms what is going to be covered during which session.

Ask the students to explain how they ended up doing Reiki in the first place, what they have been doing with their Reiki since they learned it, and what has prompted them to move on to Master level.

Reiju empowerment

Talk the students through Hatsurei ho, culminating in you giving them all a Master level empowerment (using the empowerment Kotodama): once they have been doing Seishin Toitsu for a while you ask them to keep their hands in gassho and you go round giving Reiju.

When it's their turn, rest your hand on their shoulder as an indication that they can stop doing the visualisation and just be still to receive their empowerment.

Obtain feedback on their experiences.

The Original System

Give a brief overview of Usui's original system and what was taught at each level, so that this course and its content can be seen in context.

The original system was a self-healing and spiritual development system, not a treatment technique, and the various energies that you learned to work with were there because of what they would do for you in terms of your self-healing and spiritual development, not because of any treatment benefits.

Usui's system was a path to enlightenment that involved personal commitment to work with the exercises long-term and to reap the benefits of one's efforts.

Experiencing Energies

Explain that energies can be experienced in different ways. They can be experienced using symbols, using chanting, and using intent. These three areas will be covered on the course.

Students have already used CKR and SHK to experience the energies of earth ki and heavenly ki, and these symbols elicit these energies whether or not the student has been 'attuned' to the symbols – whatever that means.

Though the common belief within the world of Reiki is that the symbols won't work for you – they are useless – unless you have been specifically attuned to them, this is not the case.

For a long time the only way that people knew how to connect you to the energy was by using an attunement, so nobody knew how to connect someone to Reiki without using symbols, to see if you really needed to be attuned to them for them to work for you.

Now from Japan have come Reiju empowerments which connect you to Reiki without symbols entering into the process, and people thus connected can use the symbols perfectly well.

Student Feedback

For two weeks before the course, students have been meditating daily on the energies of the 'Tibetan' and the Usui Master symbols.

Now they give their feedback, explaining what they have experienced. Emphasise that there is no 'right' way to experience the energies: your experience is your own and is right for you.

There may well be some similarities– sometimes striking similarities – between the students' descriptions, and at the end of this session they have now been exposed to the results of eight weeks of meditations (assuming four students on the course).

Talk about Symbols

The students have read in the manual about how the Master symbols an be used in practice, and there are other symbols in the manual for them to become familiar with, but they should not get too bogged down with symbols and when they should be used: the ideal when working with Reiki is to use symbols – or not – intuitively, going with whichever symbol (or kotodama) feels like the right thing to use at any moment... so you don't plan these things in an academic way: you get your head out of the way, don't try, don't think, just merge with the energy and let it happen.

The Kotodama

Explain a bit about the kotodama and where they came from, and how they are the original way of experiencing the energies, taught to most of Usui's students. They predate the use of symbols within Reiki.

Explain that there were three Kotodama introduced at Second Degree level, and a further one introduced at Master level. The Second Degree Kotodama are Focus, Harmony and Connection, and these are the Kotodama that we are going to be using this morning; the empowerment Kotodama comes tomorrow afternoon.

We need to consider Reiki's Buddhist connections: Buddhism is all about experiencing things as they really are, and the idea is that we are a combination of physical reality and spiritual essence.

By working with the focus and harmony kotodama over an extended period, Usui's students learned to become or assimilate the energies of earth ki and heavenly ki - to fully experience their physical reality and their spiritual essence, which is a powerful method for achieving balance.

Students would have spent 6-9 months working with the focus kotodama before spending a similar period working with the harmony kotodama.

Then some of the Second Degree students would have moved on to experience 'oneness' by using the Connection Kotodama.

Experiencing oneness was said to have been one of the goals of Usui's original system. Oneness is seen as the ultimate reality: they way things really are.

So the Kotodama are there because of what they will do for the student, not because they are useful when working on other people... though they are useful in this respect.

Kotodama Chanting

For each of the three Second Degree Kotodama, chant each one for a few minutes, all together, and then sit quietly to experience the 'ripples' that the chanting produces. Then obtain feedback.

Start by pronouncing the kotodama sound a few times so that the students are familiar with it – they have already been listening to it on their audio CD.

You are going to chant the sound yourself on your own, once, to begin with, then breathing in reasonably loudly so that the students can hear when the next one is coming, and then you all chant together on the out-breath, and breathe in together.

Do this for several minutes, and then ask the students to simply 'let the energy flow' for a few minutes.

People don't generally feel too much while they are actually chanting the sound: it is only afterwards that they will feel the distinctive 'signature' of the energy. They should notice how their body feels, notice what is going on in their head – if anything – and where there attention is.

Are they very definitely in the room or have the 'drifted off with the fairies'?

This is their first experience of earth ki, of heavenly ki, and of oneness, and if they really want to get to grips with these energies and this state then they need to chant these sounds regularly.

Most people conclude that the Kotodama give a stronger, cleaner, clearer, deeper connection to the energy when compared to the corresponding symbol.

Practical use of Kotodama

The focus and harmony Kotodama can be used as an alternative to CKR or SHK when treating, and represent the same energies. Just chant the sound – silently – to yourself either three times or endlessly as you treat, and allow the energy to flow.

There is no reason why you couldn't chant the sound out loud when you treat, but the recipient might be a little surprised if they were not expecting it!

You could use the connection Kotodama at the start of a treatment by way of helping you to 'merge' with the recipient, and to carry out distant healing you would focus your attention on the recipient – set a definite intent – chant the connection Kotodama and merge with the recipient; allow the energy to flow.

Using Kotodama on Each Other – practical exercise (optional: if you have time)

Split the students into pairs. One is on the treatment table and one sits at the head. The person sitting at the head rests their hands on either side of the temples and lets the energy flow for a while.

Then they chant the focus Kotodama silently and let the energy flow for a while. Then they chant the harmony Kotodama silently and let the energy flow for a while.

Obtain feedback, swap over, and repeat.

Conclusion to morning session

Refocus on the main theme: energies can be experienced in different ways, using symbols, chants and also using intent – to be dealt with tomorrow. Symbols are a way of representing the energies in a visual form and they will work for you whether or not you have been attuned to the symbol.

Chanting sounds – Kotodama – is another way of representing the energies, a way that was taught to most of Usui's students, and the Kotodama are there to represent two important energies and an important state that you need to get to grips with in order to further your self-healing and spiritual development, which is what Usui's system was all about.

Symbols and Kotodama can be used when treating other people, and the ideal is to use them intuitively, going with whichever symbol or kotodama wants be used on a particular occasion: no planning, no expectations, just merging with the energy and letting it happen.

The more we can 'get ourselves out of the way' and become the energy, the more intuitive impressions will come to us, and we will be exploring out intuitive potential tomorrow.

Saturday afternoon

1. Overview: Western-style attunements
2. Receive a 'Western' Master attunement.
3. Learn how to attune others 'Western' style, using Second Degree as an example.
4. Learn how to attune at Master level and First Degree level.

Guidelines

Start by explaining where Attunements come from, how there are endless variations within the world of Reiki, how the individual details don't seem to matter a great deal, how in practice they will probably choose to use Reiju certainly on any Reiki1/Reiki2 courses that they run, and that we are teaching them how to attune so that this course is compatible with other Reiki Master courses.

Give a Western Master attunement

Carry out a Western Master attunement on them.

Learning exercises

Now is their opportunity to demonstrate how much they have learned, how much they know about carrying out Second Degree attunements:

Seated exercise: split them into pairs. One person will describe to the other person all the stages of carrying out a Second Degree attunement, starting with all the individual stages of 'setting the scene', moving on to 'opening the student', 'putting the symbols in' and finishing with 'closing things down'.

The other person will listen and provide any 'hints' or suggestions or pointers that might be necessary to make sure that both of them are happy with what has been described and that no stages have been missed out.

If there are four people on the course, they can now swap partners if you like and the process is repeated, now with the person who had been listening doing the talking/describing.

As they do this, the teacher can wander round, chipping in if necessary to explain things or remind people of something they have missed.

Standing exercise: assuming there are four students, two of them stand up behind empty chairs ready to carry out attunements on the imaginary person in front of them, and the other students stand in front of the chairs, ready to give verbal instructions.

The people giving the instructions take it in turns, so student 'A' gives the instructions for 'setting the scene', student 'B' then gives the instructions for 'opening the student' etc.

Once the attunement is over the students swap over, and the ones who were previously giving the instructions get to be told by the other two what to do.

The teacher encourages, chips in, and stops the descriptions at relevant points in order to give practical suggestions.

Explain Master attunements

Now explain how to carry out Master attunements – how they differ from those at Second Degree - easy if you understand how to carry out Second Degree attunements.

Explain First Degree attunements

Now explain how to carry out the First Degree attunements – how they differ from those at Second Degree.

'Drawing' exercise

If you have time, this is nice to do. You will need a big A3 writing pad and a selection of coloured marker pens. The four students take it in turns to be the 'scribe' or 'artist' for the group.

On the first page the scribe writes 'setting the scene' at the top of the page and the other three tell the scribe what the stages are... the scribe does drawings and key words to summarise the stages.

Much hilarity can sometimes ensue depending on the drawing ability of the student!

Then the students swap round and the next student writes 'opening the student' at the top of the next fresh page, and does drawings and writes key words to summarise the main stages of this section, with the other three students telling them what the stages are, and making artistic suggestions!

Recap Master and First Degree attunements

Now you can revisit the Master and First Degree attunements, with the students telling you what the differences are between Reiki2 attunements and Master attunements, and Reiki2 attunements and Reiki1 attunements.

Sunday morning

1. Receive a Reiju empowerment at Master level.
2. Review of Day One: any questions?
3. The importance of intent: directing energy using intent/visualisation, and 'frequency setting'
4. Working with intuition: expanding our experience of Reiji ho, perceiving the chakras, and "mind's eye" visual shortcuts.

Guidelines

Start by seeing if the students have any questions or comments based on what they covered yesterday.

Ask them to tell you how a Master attunement differs from a Second Degree attunement, and how the First Degree attunements work when compared with Second Degree.

This is the last time we will mention this!

Give a Master empowerment

Go through Kenyoku and Joshin Kokkyu Ho, leading to you giving the students a Master level Reiju empowerment; get feedback.

Talk about Intent

Reiki is very simple. The energy will go where you focus your attention, whether on yourself, on other people in a treatment context, or on other people at a distance.

We have already touched on this when we used the 'many hands' method on Reiki2: you allowed your attention to dwell over a wider area and the energy followed your focus and focused itself over a wider area too.

The visualisation of hands was just a convenient shortcut to focus your intent in a particular way, and can be dispensed with.

Practical Exercise #1

The students split into pairs.

One is on the treatment table, the other sits at the head, resting the hands near the temples. They let the energy flow for a while, and then bring in imaginary hands cupping round the back of the head and hovering over the front of the face, and cocoon the head with energy for a while.

Then, keeping their hands in the same position, they take their attention away from the head and direct their attention towards the right leg, imagining that the energy travels down the energy, accumulating and building up and intensifying in the foot and lower leg.

Obtain feedback, swap over and repeat.

Intent and the Nature of the energy we are working with

Intent can also be used to govern the nature of the energy that we are working with, without needing to use a symbol or a chant to generate or connect us to a particular energy.

Practical Exercise #2

Talk the students through the 'frequency scale' meditation and obtain feedback.

Talk about Intuition

All the students on the course are intuitive, really, really intuitive. They have evidence of this because they have been working with Reiji ho.

Working with intuition is deceptively simple: all you need to do is to get your head out of the way, don't try, don't think, no expectations, just merge with the energy, bliss out on the energy and let it happen.

This state of mind comes up again and again with Reiki: on first degree I have my students disappear into the energy, merge with the energy as they treat... this is the best state of mind to have when carrying out distant healing... this is the same state of mind that you use when accessing intuitive information during Reiji ho.

Although your hands are moving when using Reiji ho, it is still you that is controlling the movements: your nerves, your muscles... intuitive information is coming through to you and being translated into muscle movements.

But intuitive information can come through in other ways, and you can set your intent to intuit different aspects of a person.: so you can use imaginary hands that drift in your mind's eye, and you can intuit areas of physical need, or mental/emotional need, or spiritual need, whether the person is in front of you on the treatment table or 1,000 miles away.

Practical exercise #3 – optional (if you have time)

Students split into pairs.

One is on the treatment table and the other stands by the side. They feel their connection to the energy and draw energy down to the Dantien, feeling the energy building up and intensifying in the Dantien.

Students carry out Reiji ho for a while if they are able to, to find the main areas of need (otherwise skip this bit and move swiftly on to the next bit...).

Now they try using imaginary hands (with their hands held in the prayer position for example, or resting over their Dantien) to see where the imaginary hands want to drift to.

Then use real/imaginary hands but with the intent that they should be guided to areas of physical need, and after a while they set their intent so they can be guided to areas of mental/emotional need.

Obtain feedback.

Talk about sensing Chakras

The students already know what is going on with their energy systems and the energy systems of the people around them. They just need to suspend their disbelief and try.

We are going to go through an exercise where the students directly experience or perceive another student's chakras.

The chakras may be perceived in different ways. There may be a visual component, there may be a sound, or a feeling, or an impression, or a combination of these, and the way that we might expect to perceive the chakras may well not be the way that we actually perceive them in practice.

Practical exercise #4

Students split into pairs.

One sits in a chair with their eyes closed and wait for their chakras to be perceived. The other student sits near them with their eyes closed ready to perceive the chakras. The 'perceiver' does this:

They feel their connection to the energy and draw energy down to the Dantien, feeling the energy building up and intensifying in the Dantien.

They focus their attention on the recipient, expand their energy to engulf the recipient and feel themselves merging or becoming one with the recipient.

They now consider the chakras.

Maybe they consider each chakra in turn for a while, before moving on to the next, after a while returning to some of the chakras to compare them... maybe they consider the chakras from afar, noticing if some chakras attract or draw their attention.

How do the chakras seem? Which ones need attention in terms of needing Reiki to help them to be in a better state for the recipient? Which chakras – although maybe bigger or smaller than others – give a sense of being ok for the recipient?

Obtain feedback.

Accept the impressions that the student provides. Emphasise that a particular chakra state may be appropriate for the recipient, and that they should not be worried if a particular chakra seems more closed down, for example.

This should change with time, and with working with Reiki regularly, or may simply be fine for them. We wouldn't want to impose our blueprint for 'balanced chakras' but need to be guided by our impression of which chakras require attention to be directed towards them.

The students will be surprised to find that they can get a sense of what is going on with the recipients' chakras, and the descriptions and impressions they receive are likely to be different from each other.

Swap over and repeat.

Visual shortcuts

Intuitive information is intuitive information, and this can come through to us in many ways. We can if we wish set up a 'constructed' visual method to access intuitive information.

Here is such an example: use a 'mixing desk' with seven 'sliders' that move along a scale from −100 via zero to +100. Each slider represents a chakra.

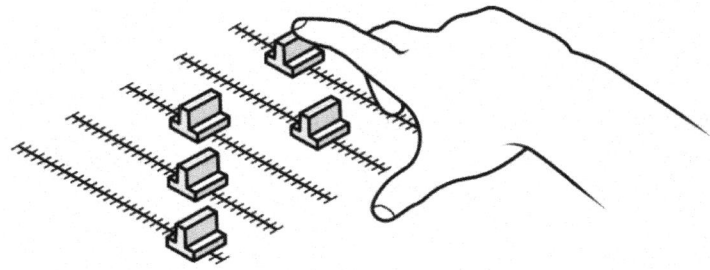

Focus your attention on a chakra and 'look' at its slider. If it hovers in the middle then the chakra is balanced, if it drifts down the scale then the chakra is moving sluggishly/closed down to the extent that the slider drifts down the scale, and if the slider moves up the scale then the chakra is spinning too fast.

Interestingly, you can even use such a constructed visual image to focus your intent: by 'pushing' on a slider you can help to bring a chakra into balance... thus the constructed visual image can be used both to focus the energy using intent, and to give feedback as to what is happening with the recipient.

Conclusion to morning session

This section has been all about moving beyond self-imposed limitations, to see what is possible when we suspend our disbelief and simply have a go.

We are not suggesting that you routinely carry out all these various exercises all the time when you treat – Reiki should be a simple and clutter-free practice after all - and we have gone through these exercises to show students what they can do, to open their eyes to some of the possibilities.

The possibilities are endless.

The exciting proposition is to use intent and intuition together: to focus the energy using intent, while being guided intuitively.

Sunday afternoon

1. Receive a Reiju empowerment.
2. Learn how to carry our Reiju empowerments and practice on each other.
3. Learn how Reiju can be use at different levels and practice on each other.
4. The benefits of Reiju
5. Distant connections
6. The empowerment Kotodama
7. Learn how to empower yourself.
8. Conclusion

Guidelines

Start by explaining what Usui did to empower people and where empowerments come from, and emphasise their elegance and simplicity when compared with Western attunements.

Give Reiju

Now carry out 'plain' empowerments on all the students, while they are watching.

They all sit with their eyes open and watch you carry out the introductory stage, and when you move towards each person in turn, they put their hands into the prayer

position and close their eyes (while the others watch)...
when that empowerment is finished you move their
hands down into their lap and they open their eyes to
watch you carry out the remainder of the
empowerments... so they all get to receive one
empowerment and watch three empowerments
(assuming four students on the course).

Obtain feedback on what they felt.

Students give Demonstration

Have one student volunteer to stand up and talk
everyone through/demonstrate the introductory stage of
Reiju; you chip in with explanations and clarifications.

Now have another student volunteer to demonstrate the
individual empowerment; again, you chip in with
clarifications, explanations and practical pointers.

Reiju at First Degree

Talk about how Reiju can be carried out at First Degree
level, and have the students pair up and do First Degree
Reiju on each other; then they swap over and return the
favour.

Obtain feedback on how they feel giving and receiving.

Important points:

- Intent is that the recipient should be permanently connected to Reiki, that they should receive what they need.
- We do three of these on our Reiki1 courses because it's nice to do a few and three fits in nicely with the schedule.
- These 'plain' empowerments can be carried out at Reiki shares.

Reiju at Second Degree

Talk about how Reiju can be carried out at Second Degree level, and have the students pair up and perform "Focus" Reiju on each other; then they swap over and return the favour.

Obtain feedback on how they feel giving and receiving.

Important points:

- Many students experience "Reiju+Kotodama" as more intense than 'plain' Reiju, and quite often the empowerment has a particular flavour that echoes he student's experience when working with the corresponding Kotodama.
- There would obviously be three empowerments carried out at Second Degree level.

Reiju at Master Level

Talk about how Reiju can be used at Master level: by using the empowerment Kotodama.

Benefits of Reiju

Talk about the benefits of Reiju when compared with western attunements.

Distant Connections and Self-empowerments

Talk about ways of carrying out distant attunements and empowerments, and ways of empowering yourself. You then take a detour via the empowerment Kotodama before describing the energy-ball self-empowerment method.

The Empowerment Kotodama

Lead students through chanting the empowerment Kotodama and experiencing its energy; get feedback.

The Energy-Ball Self-Empowerment

Now describe the energy-ball self-empowerment method, and talk the students through kenyoku/joshin kokkyu ho/energy ball; get feedback and bask in the smiles of the students!

Conclusion to the course

Remind the students of the main areas that they have covered, and the main principles/themes that have come through the course.

Remind them of the simplicity of the original system and the focus on self-development and self-healing.

Make suggestions for further work that they can do.

Reiki Master Homework

The important thing now is to make a regular part of your life, and here is my prescription for success with Reiki at this level:

- Hatsurei every day, finishing with the energy-ball self empowerment
- Get to grips with the Hara defining exercise and practise it for at least 6 months
- Get to grips with the energies of the Kotodama by chanting them regularly. Spend 3-6 months working with each one, in this order: focus, harmony, connection
- Develop your use of intuition and intent through regular practice. Experiment to see what's possible.
- Explore mindfulness, and live Usui Sensei's precepts

TEACHING REIKI AT EVENING CLASS

Introduction

I was asked to provide evening classes at Sawston Village College in Cambridgeshire, and Tuesday 25th September 2001 saw the first session of a ten-week Reiki practitioner course, covering Reiki First and Second Degrees.

I limited myself to teaching a group of 12 students on the evening class, and the course proved so popular that the College had a waiting list of 25 people for the new course that started in January 2002!

I no longer run evening classes, but it was a wonderful adventure, and lovely to be able to echo more the original way of teaching Reiki: over a longer period of time rather than in a couple of days.

I found that the students built up a lovely sense of community as they progressed together.

For the benefit of any Masters who are thinking of teaching Reiki at evening class, I have put together a complete guide to teaching Reiki in this way, with First and Second Degree taught over 10 weekly sessions.

In this guide you will find an overview of the course, showing:

1. What I covered on each session
2. What I spoke about
3. What the students learned
4. What practical exercises they went through during each evening
5. What their handout contained
6. What homework they were given

I also included the text of ten A4 sheets that I used as weekly handouts.

Each sheet encapsulates what was done on that evening. It:

1. Gives the essential points of the information that was imparted
2. Recaps the practical exercises they were given
3. Provides them with some homework to carry out

Finally, I have included suggestions as to how you can structure each evening class session, giving examples from my notes.

If you wish, you can use the enclosed handouts on your own evening classes, or use them as a guide to help you develop your own materials.

Here's a summary of what happened during each weekly session:

Session One

Talk about these topics	What is Reiki: history and background
Students learn these aspects	Kenyoku & Joshin Kokkyu ho
Students practice these exercises	Kenyoku & Joshin Kokkyu ho Play with energy
Handout deals with this	What is Reiki? Kenyoku & Joshin Kokkyu ho
Homework consists of this	Kenyoku & Joshin Kokkyu ho Feel energy fields

Session Two

Talk about these topics	Effects of attunements & self-treatments
Students learn these aspects	Usui self-treatment meditation Hatsurei ho
Students practice these exercises	Usui self-treatment meditation Hatsurei ho
Handout deals with this	Effects of attunements & self-treatments Usui self-treatment meditation Hatsurei ho
Homework consists of this	Usui self-treatment meditation Hatsurei ho

Session Three

Talk about these topics	What it's like to give & receive Reiki
Students learn these aspects	Seated treatments Feeling the energy field Scanning
Students practice these exercises	Seated treatments Feeling the energy field Scanning
Handout deals with this	What it's like to give & receive Reiki Seated treatments Feeling the energy field Scanning
Homework consists of this	Seated treatments Feeling the energy field Scanning

Session Four

Talk about these topics	The effect of Reiki treatments
Students learn these aspects	Couch treatments
Students practice these exercises	Couch treatments Feeling the energy field Scanning
Handout deals with this	The effect of Reiki treatments Couch treatments
Homework consists of this	Couch treatments Feeling the energy field Scanning

Session Five

Talk about these topics	Summary of First Degree Making Reiki part of your life
Students learn these aspects	Western-style self-treatments
Students practice these exercises	Western-style self-treatments
Handout deals with this	Making Reiki part of your life Western-style self-treatments Second Degree symbols to learn
Homework consists of this	Western-style self-treatments Second Degree symbols to learn

Session Six

Talk about these topics	Symbols (general) CKR Intuition
Students learn these aspects	The use of symbols (general) The use of CKR Reiji ho
Students practice these exercises	Energy meditation on CKR Sending/receiving CKR energy Reiji ho
Handout deals with this	The use of symbols (general) The use of CKR Reiji ho
Homework consists of this	Energy meditation using CKR Reiji ho

Session Seven

Talk about these topics	Symbols: SHK
Students learn these aspects	The use of SHK
Students practice these exercises	Energy meditation on SHK Sending/receiving SHK energy Reiji ho
Handout deals with this	The use of SHK More on intuition
Homework consists of this	Energy meditation using SHK Reiji ho

Session Eight

Talk about these topics	Symbols: HSZSN
Students learn these aspects	Distant healing methods
Students practice these exercises	Energy meditation using HSZSN Distant healing Reiji ho
Handout deals with this	Distant healing
Homework consists of this	Energy meditation using HSZSN Distant healing Reiji ho

Session Nine

Talk about these topics	Boosting the flow of energy when you treat
Students learn these aspects	"Many hands" technique Use of the Hui Yin
Students practice these exercises	"Many hands" technique Hui Yin method
Handout deals with this	"Many hands" technique The Hui Yin method
Homework consists of this	"Many hands" technique The Hui Yin method

Session Ten

Talk about these topics	The power of intent
Students learn these aspects	Eye technique Breath technique Moving energy with intent
Students practice these exercises	Eye technique Breath technique Moving energy with intent
Handout deals with this	The power of intent Eye technique Breath technique Moving energy with intent
Homework consists of this	Eye technique Breath technique Moving energy with intent

First and Second Degree in 10 A4 hand-outs

In the following pages you can see the text of the ten A4 handouts that I used for these evening classes.

Well, there were actually eleven sheets: after week five (when they had completed First Degree) also gave them a sheet with the three Reiki symbols on it, so they could start learning them before they came along for t heir five Second Degree sessions.

I have included a few facsimiles of the actual handouts so you can see how they were laid out.

Each hand-out has two vertical columns. It is surprising how much information you can provide in such a small amount of space if you really try!

Why not use these as the basis for your own.

You can download the originals for free here:

www.reiki-evolution.co.uk/eveningclass.pdf

Week 1

What is Reiki?

In its original Japanese form, Reiki was a path to enlightenment, and part of that path was to do energy work on yourself and on others. In Western Reiki, the focus has been more on the 'healing' aspects of the system.

You can see Reiki as an oriental version of spiritual healing: you channel an unlimited source of healing energy for your benefit and the benefit of people that you treat.

You can see the energy as Divine light or Divine love, or you can view the energy as 'chi': the energy that underlies such things as acupuncture, tai chi, shiatsu and feng shui.

Mikao Usui (1865-1926) developed Reiki in the early part of the 20th century, and Reiki draws on lots of existing oriental traditions that were present in Japan at the time:

1. Traditional Japanese Hand Healing ('teate')
2. Energy Cultivation Techniques
3. Martial Arts
4. Shintoism
5. Mikkyo (mystical) Buddhism

Usui, a Tendai Buddhist, was well versed in all the above areas, and their healing potential. He studied voraciously, not only Western medical ideas, but also ancient texts, and he was involved in a high-level psychic/clairvoyant development group. His search for the ultimate purpose of life led him to fast and meditate on Mt Kurama, near Kyoto, and a moment of enlightenment contributed to the development of Reiki.

Usui was a famous healer in his lifetime, teaching thousands of people in Japan. Reiki's journey to the West was through one of Usui's less experienced Masters students - a retired surgeon commander from the Imperial Navy called Dr Chujiro Hayashi - and through one of Hayashi's Master students - Mrs Hawayo Takata.

Dr Hayashi emphasised the healing side of Reiki rather than the 'spiritual path', and Mrs Takata simplified things for a Western audience, including making up a story about Usui being a Christian theologian. This was done in order to make a Japanese healing technique acceptable to a hostile American public after WWII.

Energy Exercises

Here are two simple energy exercises from the original Japanese form of Reiki.

Kenyoku ('Dry Bathing' or 'Brushing Off') to get rid of negative energy.

Rest your right hand on your left shoulder/upper chest, and as you exhale run your hand down your torso to your right hip. Now do this with your left hand (starting on your right shoulder), and finally repeat with the right hand again.

Now you are going to brush along your arms. Start with the right hand on the left shoulder. As you exhale, brush along the outside of your left arm and past your fingertips, exhaling as you do so. Do this with your left hand on your right arm, and then finish by repeating with the right hand again.

Joshin Kokkyu Ho ('Soul Cleansing Breathing Method') to balance and boost your energy.

Put your hands on your lap with your palms facing upwards and breathe naturally through your nose. Focus on your Dantien point and relax. Dantien is an energy centre two finger-breadths below your tummy button and one third of the way into your body.

When you breathe in, visualise energy or light flooding into your crown and passing through your body into your Dantien. As you pause before exhaling, feel that energy expand throughout your body, melting all your tensions. When you breathe out, imagine that the energy floods out of your body in all directions as far as infinity. Repeat for at least 3 minutes.

Homework

This week I would like you carry out Kenyoku/Joshin Kokkyu Ho every day - religiously - at least once a day for 5 minutes in total. If you can, do it three times a day.

I would also like you to practice feeling energy fields: on yourself (between your hands and over your body), on your family and friends, on your pets, on your houseplants.

Week 1 – Column 1

What is Reiki ?

In its original Japanese form, Reiki was a path to enlightenment, and part of that path was to do energy work on yourself and on others. In Western Reiki, the focus has been more on the 'healing' aspects of the system.

You can see Reiki as an oriental version of spiritual healing: you channel an unlimited source of healing energy for your benefit and the benefit of people that you treat.

You can see the energy as Divine light or Divine love, or you can view the energy as 'chi': the energy that underlies such things as acupuncture, tai chi, shiatsu and feng shui.

Mikao Usui (1865-1926) developed Reiki in the early part of the 20th century, and Reiki draws on lots of existing oriental traditions that were present in Japan at the time:

1.   Traditional Japanese Hand Healing ('teate')
2.   Energy Cultivation Techniques
3.   Martial Arts
4.   Shintoism
5.   Mikkyo (mystical) Buddhism

Usui, a Tendai Buddhist, was well versed in all the above areas, and their healing potential. He studied voraciously, not only Western medical ideas, but also ancient texts, and he was involved in a high-level psychic/clairvoyant development group. His search for the ultimate purpose of life led him to fast and meditate on Mt Kurama, near Kyoto, and a moment of enlightenment contributed to the development of Reiki.

Usui was a famous healer in his lifetime, teaching thousands of people in Japan. Reiki's journey to the West was through one of Usui's less experienced Masters students - a retired surgeon commander from the Imperial Navy called Dr Chujiro Hayashi - and through one of Hayashi's Master students - Mrs Hawayo Takata.

Dr Hayashi emphasised the healing side of Reiki rather than the 'spiritual path', and Mrs Takata simplified things for a Western audience, including making up a story about Usui being a Christian theologian. This was done in order to make a Japanese healing technique acceptable to a hostile American public after WWII.

Week 1 – Column 2

Energy Exercises

Here are two simple energy exercises from the original Japanese form of Reiki.

Kenyoku ('Dry Bathing' or 'Brushing Off') to get rid of negative energy.

Rest your right hand on your left shoulder/upper chest, and as you exhale run your hand down your torso to your right hip. Now do this with your left hand (starting on your right shoulder), and finally repeat with the right hand again.

Now you are going to brush along your arms. Start with the right hand on the left shoulder. As you exhale, brush along the outside of your left arm and past your fingertips, exhaling as you do so. Do this with your left hand on your right arm, and then finish by repeating with the right hand again.

Joshin Kokkyu Ho ('Soul Cleansing Breathing Method') to balance and boost your energy.

Put your hands on your lap with your palms facing upwards and breathe naturally through your nose. Focus on your Dantien point and relax. Dantien is an energy centre two finger-breadths below your tummy button and one third of the way into your body.

When you breathe in, visualise energy or light flooding into your crown and passing through your body into your Dantien. As you pause before exhaling, feel that energy expand throughout your body, melting all your tensions. When you breathe out, imagine that the energy floods out of your body in all directions as far as infinity. Repeat for at least 3 minutes.

Homework

This week I would like you carry out Kenyoku/Joshin Kokkyu Ho every day - religiously - at least once a day for 5 minutes in total. If you can, do it three times a day.

I would also like you to practice feeling energy fields: on yourself (between your hands and over your body), on your family and friends, on your pets, on your houseplants.

Week 2

What will Reiki do for me ?

Reiki makes most people feel: more calm, content and serene; more laid back; more positive and better able to cope; less stressed and hassled by people/situations. Usually this builds up gradually, and you'll notice the changes with hindsight.

Once you've been attuned, the energy starts to work on you straight away, and sometimes this can bring things to the surface, e.g. emotional ups and downs, physical symptoms (like a cold), or a feeling of general dissatisfaction for a while. This shows that things are being released and brought into balance.

When people say that Reiki has changed their life, it is usually because Reiki has helped give people a sense of clarity: Reiki helps you to work out what things really are important in your life, and gives you a kick up the backside to make what changes are necessary. It can also enhance your spirituality.

Sometimes being attuned to Reiki can eliminate physical and emotional problems very quickly, for example long-term back pain, and over time can enhance psychic/clairvoyant abilities

Hatsu Rei Ho: Energy Exercises
('Start up Reiki technique')

Start
Hands in your lap, palms down. Focus on Dantien and say 'I'm starting Hatsurei now' to subconscious.
Kenyoku - see prev. handout
Connect to Reiki
Hold your palms up to the sky and imagine energy flooding through your hands from above, down to your Dantien.
Joshin Kokkyu Ho - 3 mins; see prev. handout
Gassho - 3 mins at least
Simply put your hands into the 'prayer' position and focus on the point where your middle fingers touch.
Seishin Toitsu - 3 mins at least
Hands in the prayer position. When you breathe in, pull energy through your hands and take the energy to your Dantien. Feel the energy get stronger and when you breathe out, flood the energy out of your hands again. Repeat.
Finish
Hands back to your lap, palms down. Say 'I'm finishing Hatsurei now' to subconscious. Open eyes and shake hands up & down/side to side.

Self-Treatment Meditation

1. Sit comfortably on a chair; eyes closed.
2. Imagine a carbon copy of you sitting in front of you, with its back towards you.
3. Imagine that you are treating yourself, by resting your imaginary hands in a series of imaginary hand positions on the head.
4. Imagine yourself holding each position for about 3-6 minutes.
5. Focus on imagining yourself channelling Reiki through your hands into 'you'.

As you do this, you may feel 'hands' on your head. If it is simpler for you, you can imagine an 'imaginary you' standing up behind you and sending Reiki into the five hand positions.

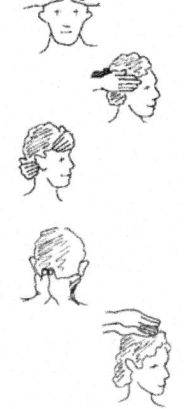

Homework

This week I would like you carry out Hatsu Rei Ho for 12-15 minutes a day, without fail.

I would also like you to practice the Usui Self-Treatment meditation for 15-25 minutes a day, again without fail.

Week 2 – Column 1

What will Reiki do for me ?

Reiki makes most people feel: more calm, content and serene; more laid back; more positive and better able to cope; less stressed and hassled by people/situations. Usually this builds up gradually, and you'll notice the changes with hindsight.

Once you've been attuned, the energy starts to work on you straight away, and sometimes this can bring things to the surface, e.g. emotional ups and downs, physical symptoms (like a cold), or a feeling of general dissatisfaction for a while. This shows that things are being released and brought into balance.

When people say that Reiki has changed their life, it is usually because Reiki has helped give people a sense of clarity: Reiki helps you to work out what things really are important in your life, and gives you a kick up the backside to make what changes are necessary. It can also enhance your spirituality.

Sometimes being attuned to Reiki can eliminate physical and emotional problems very quickly, for example long-term back pain, and over time can enhance psychic/clairvoyant abilities

Hatsu Rei Ho: Energy Exercises

('Start up Reiki technique')

Start

Hands in your lap, palms down. Focus on Dantien and say 'I'm starting Hatsurei now' to subconscious.

Kenyoku - see prev. handout

Connect to Reiki

Hold your palms up to the sky and imagine energy flooding through your hands from above, down to your Dantien.

Joshin Kokkyu Ho - 3 mins; see prev. handout

Gassho - 3 mins at least

Simply put your hands into the 'prayer' position and focus on the point where your middle fingers touch.

Seishin Toitsu - 3 mins at least

Hands in the prayer position. When you breathe in, pull energy through your hands and take the energy to your Dantien. Feel the energy get stronger and when you breathe out, flood the energy out of your hands again. Repeat.

Finish

Hands back to your lap, palms down. Say 'I'm finishing Hatsurei now' to subconscious. Open eyes and shake hands up & down/side to side.

Week 2 – Column 2

Self-Treatment Meditation

1. Sit comfortably on a chair; eyes closed.
2. Imagine a carbon copy of you sitting in front of you, with its back towards you.
3. Imagine that you are treating yourself, by resting your imaginary hands in a series of imaginary hand positions on the head.
4. Imagine yourself holding each position for about 3-6 minutes.
5. Focus on imagining yourself channelling Reiki through your hands into 'you'.

As you do this, you may feel 'hands' on your head. If it is simpler for you, you can imagine an 'imaginary you' standing up behind you and sending Reiki into the five hand positions.

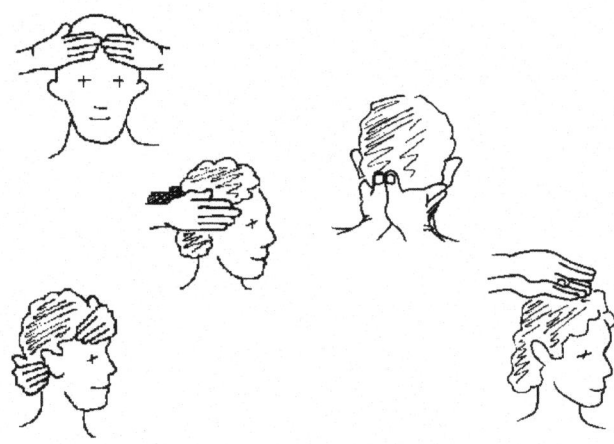

Homework

This week I would like you carry out Hatsu Rei Ho for 12-15 minutes a day, without fail.

I would also like you to practice the Usui Self-Treatment meditation for 15-25 minutes a day, again without fail.

Week 3

Giving and Receiving Reiki

Receiving Reiki

Most people feel these things: deep, deep relaxation, heat from your hands, and sometimes coloured lights. Other sensations might be floating/sinking, having no body, limbs of stone, or tingles in various places. It is a relaxing and pleasurable experience!

An 'emotional release' is quite common, which is a flood of pure emotion, a necessary stage on the way to achieving emotional balance. Sometimes aches and pains can intensify for a while during the treatment.

Giving Reiki

Most Reiki people feel heat, tingling, fizzing, buzzing, or pulsing in parts of their hands as the energy flows. With practice you can feel when the energy is flowing more and less strongly.

Some people feel mainly heat, some mainly fizzing/tingling, and some people have quite unusual sensations! What will yours be? Occasionally your hands can ache, and you might feel a bit queasy once in a blue moon, but it's only temporary!

Feel the Energy field

Feel the energy field around the body. Are there areas where it's very close to the body? Those areas are depleted. Boost them with Reiki, imagining that the energy is flooding through your hands into the aura, and then check again. Do this until the energy field is nice and even; a nice way to start off a treatment.

Scan the Body

Get the lie of the land: hover one hand over the body and as you move it, see if you can detect areas that are pulling more energy. You will end up spending more time there when you do the hands-on treatment. Doing this can help you decide on additional hand positions. Compare both knees, ankles, hips etc. Is one pulling more energy?

Scan at the end of the treatment to see whether the 'hotspots' are as 'hot' as they were at the start.

Seated Reiki Treatments

Tune yourself in to the recipient.
Intend that the treatment is for 'highest good'.
Connect to Reiki (see 'Hatsurei' instructions).

Practice feeling the person's energy field.
Scan the body to find 'hotspots'.

Start treating the shoulders.
Boost the flow of Reiki by 'drawing energy down' through your crown and out of your hands.
For the head, use the 'Usui' hand positions that you have been using in your self-treatment meditation.
Move on to the torso as follows, kneeling as necessary.

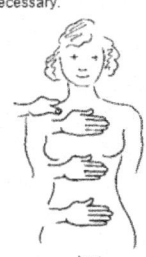

Then treat the hips, knees, and ankles.
Finish by smoothing down the energy field.
Do a little ritual that means 'I've disconnected'.

Homework

Please carry on with your daily Hatsurei and your Self-treatment meditation.

This week I would like you to carry out a seated Reiki treatment on someone each day for at least 30 minutes. This can be on the same person if necessary, but if you can find a few different people to practice on, that would be better.

When you treat someone, practice feeling their energy field and balancing their aura. Practice scanning them at the beginning and at the end of the treatment. This will help to build up the sensitivity in your hands.

Week 3 – Column 1

Giving and Receiving Reiki

Receiving Reiki

Most people feel these things: deep, deep relaxation, heat from your hands, and sometimes coloured lights. Other sensations might be floating/sinking, having no body, limbs of stone, or tingles in various places. It is a relaxing and pleasurable experience!

An 'emotional release' is quite common, which is a flood of pure emotion, a necessary stage on the way to achieving emotional balance. Sometimes aches and pains can intensify for a while during the treatment.

Giving Reiki

Most Reiki people feel heat, tingling, fizzing, buzzing, or pulsing in parts of their hands as the energy flows. With practice you can feel when the energy is flowing more and less strongly.

Some people feel mainly heat, some mainly fizzing/tingling, and some people have quite unusual sensations! What will yours be? Occasionally your hands can ache, and you might feel a bit queasy once in a blue moon, but it's only temporary!

Feel the Energy field

Feel the energy field around the body. Are there areas where it's very close to the body? Those areas are depleted. Boost them with Reiki, imagining that the energy is flooding through your hands into the aura, and then check again. Do this until the energy field is nice and even; a nice way to start off a treatment.

Scan the Body

Get the lie of the land: hover one hand over the body and as you move it, see if you can detect areas that are pulling more energy. You will end up spending more time there when you do the hands-on treatment. Doing this can help you decide on additional hand positions. Compare both knees, ankles, hips etc. Is one pulling more energy?

Scan at the end of the treatment to see whether the 'hotspots' are as 'hot' as they were at the start.

Week 3 – Column 2

Seated Reiki Treatments

Tune yourself in to the recipient.
Intend that the treatment is for 'highest good'.
Connect to Reiki (see 'Hatsurei' instructions).

Practice feeling the person's energy field.
Scan the body to find 'hotspots'.

Start treating the shoulders.
Boost the flow of Reiki by 'drawing energy down'
through your crown and out of your hands.
For the head, use the 'Usui' hand positions that you
have been using in your self-treatment meditation.
Move on to the torso as follows, kneeling as necessary.

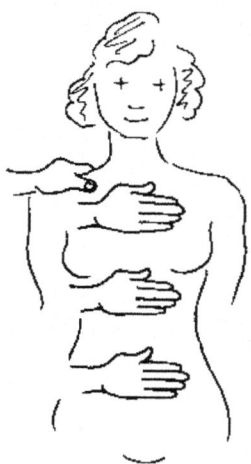

Then treat the hips, knees, and ankles.
Finish by smoothing down the energy field.
Do a little ritual that means 'I've disconnected'.

Homework

Please carry on with your daily Hatsurei and your Self-treatment meditation.

This week I would like you to carry out a seated Reiki treatment on someone each day for at least 30 minutes. This can be on the same person if necessary, but if you can find a few different people to practice on, that would be better.

When you treat someone, practice feeling their energy field and balancing their aura. Practice scanning them at the beginning and at the end of the treatment. This will help to build up the sensitivity in your hands.

Week 4

Week 4 – Column 1

Effects of Reiki Treatments

General

The effects of Reiki treatments build up cumulatively. After one treatment, most people will notice some change, but it will fizzle out after a few days usually. By repeating the exposure to Reiki at weekly intervals you build momentum and start to produce some long-term changes, without the need to keep coming back for 'top-up' visits.

At least 4-6 sessions are usually needed to make long-term changes that will 'stick'.

You cannot overdose on Reiki, so if you want to treat someone every day, then that's fine. Any strong reaction that they might have will be intensified though.

'The Reiki Effect'

Reiki makes most people feel: more calm, content and serene; more laid back; more positive and better able to cope; less stressed and hassled by people/situations. This is what many people notice after a few Reiki treatments, no matter what their specific problems.

Physical Effects

Reiki seems to work well with long-term pain, for example back pain, arthritis & rheumatism, post-operative pain, sports injuries: inflammatory pain. It can also make a real difference to low energy levels.

Anecdotally, Reiki has done some amazing things, even with very serious and even life-threatening conditions, but there is no hard scientific evidence to back up such claims.

Mental/Emotional Effects

Reiki seems to work well with stress, tension and anxiety, and sleeplessness - even if this has continued for a long time. It can deal with low spirits and depression, as well as helping with more deep-seated problems like anorexia and addiction, and low self-esteem. It will deal with suppressed grief and long-term emotional imbalances: the unresolved issues and emotional blocks that we keep a lid on, even if these date back to childhood.

Week 4 – Column 2

Couch Reiki Treatments

Tune yourself in to the recipient.
Intend that the treatment is for 'highest good'.
Connect to Reiki (see 'Hatsurei' instructions).

Practice feeling the person's energy field.
Scan the body to find 'hotspots'.

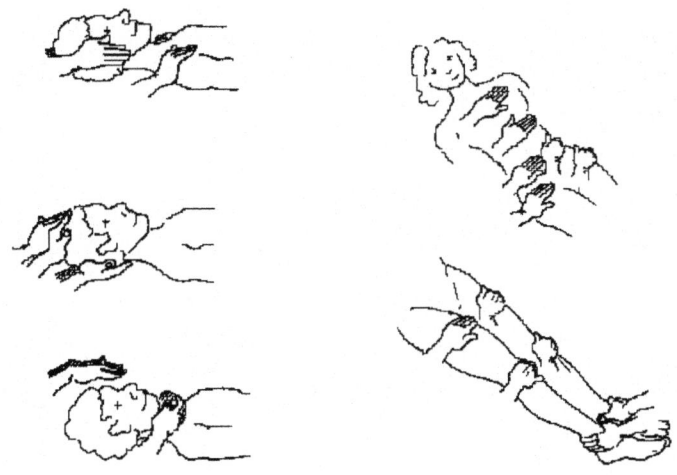

Treat shoulders for about 10 minutes.
Then the temples and crown.
Then back of head, front of face, and throat.

On the torso treat heart/solar plexus, navel and hips. Treat the thighs, knees and ankles.

Finish by smoothing down the energy field from the crown towards the ankles..
Do a little ritual that means 'I've disconnected'.

Homework

Please carry on with your daily Hatsurei and your Self-treatment meditation.

This week I would like you to carry out a supine Reiki treatment on someone each day for at least 30 minutes. This can be on the same person if necessary, but if you can find a few different people to practice on, that would be better. If you can do some 'full' hour-long treatments then that will be excellent.

Carry on feeling the energy field and doing your scanning. Your hands will become more sensitive to the energy if you do this often.

Week 5

Make Reiki a part of your Life

Recipe for Success

To gain the greatest benefits from your Reiki, you need to expose yourself to the energy on a regular basis. Here is my recipe for Reiki success:

1. Do Hatsurei every day without fail. Make it a daily routine that you carry out at the same time, like brushing your teeth.
2. Perform the Usui self-treatment meditation regularly. This is ideal to do when you are sitting in a train or a car, or even during your lunch-break!
3. Get your hands on other people. This will help you to be a strong channel, it will boost your confidence, and your sensitivity to the energy will develop.
4. Follow Usui's 'Reiki Precepts':

   Just for today,
   do not anger,
   do not worry
   Be humble (remind yourself of your many blessings)
   Be honest in your dealings with people
   Be compassionate towards yourself & others

Hand Positions: what they mean

Sometimes when you hold a hand position, you will feel more energy coming through. This can tie in with things that are going on with the person that you are treating. For example....

Shoulders: Stress and tension
Temples: Busy Mind, unable to Sleep because of many thoughts
Crown: Headaches or Low Spirits, but not always
Throat: Communication Issues: holding back and not opening up to the people close to you
Heart & Solar Plexus: Emotional centres, with S.P. tying in with more long-term unresolved issues.

Feeling a 'Hotspot' doesn't mean you are detecting disease necessarily. Reiki will support natural physiological processes like digestion, ovulation, menstruation, and support natural repairs to muscles and joints damaged through exercise.

Don't get in the frame of mind of thinking "what have you got wrong here?" when you feel something! You don't diagnose with Reiki.

'Western' Self-Treatments

Place your hands in a series of hand-positions on your body. Draw energy down from above to boost the flow of Reiki, if you wish.

Treat the shoulders, temples and crown.
Treat the back of the head and the front of the face. Treat the throat.
Move on to the heart/solar plexus, navel, and hips.

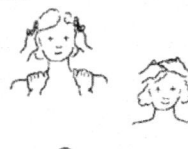

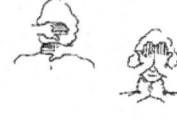

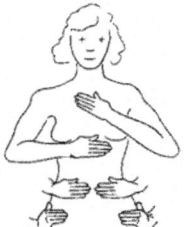

Homework

Learn the Reiki Symbols ready for next week.

Please carry on with your daily Hatsurei.

Carry out a 30 minute Western-style self-treatment every day. How does it feel?

Practice treating others, either seated or supine.

Week 5 – Column 1

Make Reiki a part of your Life

Recipe for Success

To gain the greatest benefits from your Reiki, you need to expose yourself to the energy on a regular basis. Here is my recipe for Reiki success:

1. Do Hatsurei every day without fail. Make it a daily routine that you carry out at the same time, like brushing your teeth.
2. Perform the Usui self-treatment meditation regularly. This is ideal to do when you are sitting in a train or a car, or even during your lunch-break!
3. Get your hands on other people. This will help you to be a strong channel, it will boost your confidence, and your sensitivity to the energy will develop.
4. Follow Usui's 'Reiki Precepts':

Just for today,
do not anger,
do not worry
Be humble (remind yourself of your many blessings)
Be honest in your dealings with people
Be compassionate towards yourself & others
Hand Positions: what they mean

Sometimes when you hold a hand position, you will feel more energy coming through. This can tie in with things that are going on with the person that you are treating. For example…

Shoulders: Stress and tension
Temples: Busy Mind, unable to Sleep because of many thoughts
Crown: Headaches or Low Spirits, but not always
Throat: Communication Issues: holding back and not opening up to the people close to you
Heart & Solar Plexus: Emotional centres, with S.P. tying in with more long-term unresolved issues.

Feeling a 'Hotspot' doesn't mean you are detecting disease necessarily. Reiki will support natural physiological processes like digestion, ovulation, menstruation, and support natural repairs to muscles and joints damaged through exercise.

Don't get in the frame of mind of thinking "what have you got wrong here?" when you feel something! You don't diagnose with Reiki.

Week 5 – Column 2

'Western' Self-Treatments

Place your hands in a series of hand-positions on your body. Draw energy down from above to boost the flow of Reiki, if you wish.

Treat the shoulders, temples and crown.

Treat the back of the head and the front of the face. Treat the throat.

Move on to the heart/solar plexus, navel, and hips.

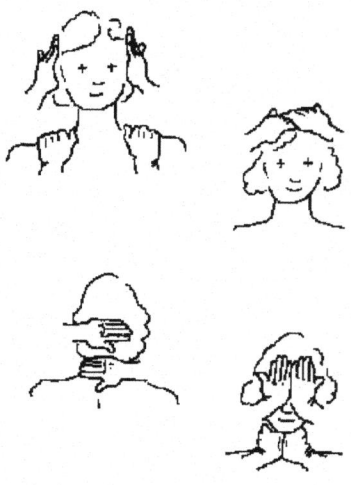

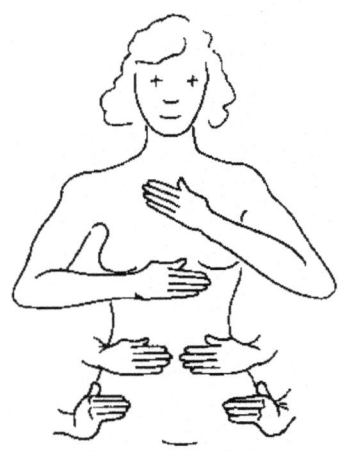

Homework

Learn the Reiki Symbols ready for next week.

Please carry on with your daily Hatsurei.

Carry out a 30 minute Western-style self-treatment every day. How does it feel?

Practice treating others, either seated or supine.

Handout for before Second Degree

The Reiki Symbols

Here are some symbols for you to look at and practice drawing. We will be using them on the Reiki Second Degree Course that starts next week, so you need to have learned them before the appropriate week. Each symbol has a name that you need to learn, and you can see the 'pronunciation guide' below. To practice drawing out the symbols, draw the lines in the order of the little arrows.

Cho Ku Rei (the spiral) is covered on week six
Cho, as in 'show'   Ku, as in 'koo'   Rei, as in 'ray'

Sei He Ki (the one with two bumps) is covered on week seven
Sei, as in 'say'   He, as in 'hay'   Ki, as in 'key'

Hon Sha Ze Sho Nen (the long, daunting one) is covered on week eight, so start practising!
Hon   rhymes with 'gone', 'on'
Sha, as in 'shah'
Ze, as in 'zay', rhymes with 'day', 'hay'
Sho, as in 'show'
Nen rhymes with 'men', 'when', 'hen'

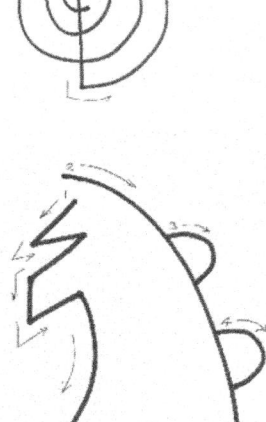

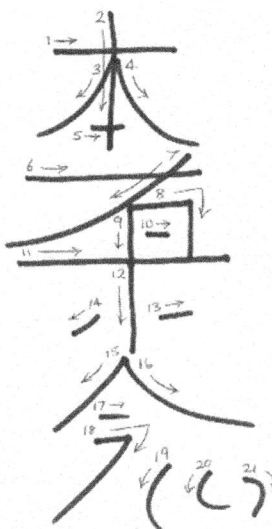

Text of the extra "Symbols" handout

The Reiki Symbols

Here are some symbols for you to look at and practice drawing. We will be using them on the Reiki Second Degree Course that starts next week, so you need to have learned them before the appropriate week. Each symbol has a name that you need to learn, and you can see the 'pronunciation guide' below. To practice drawing out the symbols, draw the lines in the order of the little arrows.

Cho Ku Rei (the spiral) is covered on week six
Cho, as in 'show', Ku, as in 'koo', Rei, as in 'ray'

Sei He Ki (the one with two bumps) is covered on week seven
Sei, as in 'say', He, as in 'hay', Ki, as in 'key'

Hon Sha Ze Sho Nen (the long, daunting one) is covered on week eight, so start practising!
Hon   rhymes with 'gone', 'on'
Sha, as in 'shah'
Ze, as in 'zay', rhymes with 'day', 'hay'
Sho, as in 'show'
Nen rhymes with 'men', 'when', 'hen'

Week 6

The week 6 hand-out is not interesting in terms of layout. It simply displays two columns with headings and text, so I have not included an image of it.

Week 6 – Column 1

The Reiki Symbols

General

The First two symbols are used routinely when giving treatments. Draw them out in the air over the back of your hand in each new hand position, and then say their name silently three times. Draw them with your fingers bunched together, with head movements, or with your eyes.

The first two symbols boost the flow of energy and focus the energy on either physical healing or mental/emotional balancing. The third symbol helps you to make a strong distant connection with someone.

CKR: Physical Healing

This symbol produces a low frequency energy that resonates at the frequency of the physical body. It enhances physical healing and the energy feels very strong in your hands. You can draw this symbol in any hand position over the body. Usui's surviving students see this energy as 'earth' energy, that reminds us of who we are.

Energy Meditation

Sit with your eyes closed and your hands in your lap, palms upwards. Imagine (draw out in your mind's eye) a big CKR above you and say its name three times. Now imagine cascades of energy/light flooding into you from the symbol, into your head, hands, torso.

How does this feel? What is distinctive about this energy? Do this for 5 minutes.

Feel CKR Energy in your Hands

You'll need someone to practice this on. 'Charge up your hands' by drawing CKR over your palm - and say its name 3 times - and then press your palms together 3 times to 'transfer the effect across' to the other hand. Then visualise a great big CKR above you - and say its name 3 times. Imagine that you are drawing down endless cascades of energy from that symbol, through your crown, through your arms, and out of your hands into the recipient.

How does this feel in your hands? What is distinctive about this energy? Do this for 5 minutes.

Week 6 – Column 2

Working with Intuition

You are already intuitive, but you probably don't know how to access this information. "Reiji Ho" ('indication of the spirit technique') allows the energy to guide your hands to the right places to treat, so instead of using standard hand positions, you gear each treatment towards the person's individual energy needs.

Close your eyes, hands in the prayer position, and imagine a strong connection to Reiki through your crown. Move your hands so they rest against your forehead and say to yourself "Please let me be guided, please let my hands be guided. Show me where to treat".

Move your hands down so they hover over the person, and make no deliberate hand movements because you will over-ride any subtle sensations and the technique won't work.

Imagine the energy flowing through your crown, shoulders, arms and hands, feel yourself joining with the energy, merging with it, becoming one with it, and allow the energy to move you hands.
Be aware of any gentle or subtle pull on your hands, and allow them to drift.

Use this method to work out where to put your hands.
Start with the shoulders for a while, use intuitive
positions on the head, and then move on to the torso,
finishing with the ankles.

The more often you deliberately make yourself open to
intuition the more definitely and consistently your hands
will move, and the faster they will move. Practice makes
perfect. Using this method will open you to other intuitive
information too, with time.

Homework

Please carry on with your daily Hatsurei.

Do an energy meditation using CKR daily. Feel the
energy flowing through your hands daily (you'll need
someone to practice this on). Become familiar with the
feel of this energy.

Practice using your intuition to guide your hands when
you treat someone, and use CKR. Do this every day for
a little while. It gets easier and easier with practice.
Practice Reiji Ho every day.

Week 7

The week 7 hand-out is not interesting in terms of layout. It simply displays two columns with headings and text, so I have not included an image of it.

Week 7 – Column 1

The Reiki Symbols

SHK: Mental/Emotional Balancing

This symbol produces a higher frequency energy than CKR. It resonates at the frequency of the thoughts and emotions. SHK enhances mental and emotional balancing and the energy feels quite gentle in your hands. You can draw this symbol over the head, heart and solar plexus. Usui's surviving students see this energy as 'celestial' energy, that produces harmony.

Keep the Symbols separate

CKR and SHK produce quite different energies, and they work best of all if you use only one energy - one symbol - in each hand position. Usui's original method of contacting the energies was to use ancient Shinto mantras, and you can only chant one mantra in your head at any one time! He kept it simple.

If you feel you need to use both energies in one hand position, use one energy for a while, take your hands away and 'brush away' that symbol, and then use the other energy. Keep them separate.

Energy Meditation

Sit with your eyes closed and your hands in your lap, palms upwards. Imagine (draw out in your mind's eye) a big SHK above you and say its name three times. Now imagine cascades of energy/light flooding into you from the symbol, into your head, hands, torso.

How does this feel? What is distinctive about this energy? Do this for 5 minutes.

Feel SHK Energy in your Hands

You'll need someone to practice this on. 'Charge up your hands' by drawing SHK over your palm - and say its name 3 times - and then press your palms together 3 times to 'transfer the effect across'. Then visualise a great big SHK above you - and say its name 3 times as usual . Imagine that you are drawing down endless cascades of energy from that symbol, through your crown, through your arms, and out of your hands into the recipient.

How does this feel in your hands? What is distinctive about this energy? Do this for 5 minutes.

Week 7 – Column 2

Giving Intense Treatments

You now have a range of different ways of approaching Reiki treatments. If you like you can do 'Reiki 1' treatments where you just let the energy flow as it likes, maybe boosting the flow of energy by drawing energy down from above.

You can make treatments more intense by drawing CKR or SHK over your hands as you move from one hand position to another. This boosts the flow of energy and gears the energy towards either physical healing or mental / emotional balancing.

The most intense way of giving a treatment is to charge your hands up with either CKR or SHK, put a big version of the symbol up in the air, and spend the whole treatment drawing energy down from that symbol. Over a course of treatments, don't use one energy to the exclusion of the other, but you can work intensely on physical healing, or mental / emotional balancing if you feel you need to.

The importance of being able to boost the flow of energy is that no-one is a perfectly clear channel for Reiki, and sometimes you cannot supply as much energy - through your clogged up energy pipework - as a part of the body needs, especially when you get to 'hot spots'. Using symbols in various ways is one way of boosting the flow of energy, coming closer to supplying the potential energy need of a part of the body.

There are other ways of boosting the flow of energy too.

Homework

Please carry on with your daily Hatsurei.

Do an energy meditation using SHK daily. Feel the energy flowing through your hands daily (you'll need someone to practice this on). Become familiar with the feel of this energy.

Now compare this energy with CKR.

Practice using your intuition to guide your hands when you treat someone, use SHK & CKR. Do this every day for a little while. It gets easier and easier with practice. Practice Reiji Ho every day.

Week 8

The week 6 hand-out is not interesting in terms of layout.

Week 8 – Column 1

Distant Healing

HSZSN: Distant Healing symbol

This is not a symbol that produces an energy of a particular frequency, but a symbol that allows the energy to be connected in a particular way: in a way where you do not need to worry about time and distance. Usui's surviving students see this symbol as producing 'oneness' within you, which allows you to transcend time and space.

Technique

The bare bones of distant healing are that you know where you want the energy to go, and you use HSZSN in some way to access that distant connection. There are several methods:

- Use a prop (doll, teddy bear, pillow, your leg), draw HSZSN over the 'prop' and Reiki it with the intention that it is the recipient.
- Imagine that you have shrunk the recipient down so that they fit in the palm of your

hand, draw HSZSN over your palm and cup the other hand over the top; send Reiki from your hands, through an 'energy tube', to the recipient.

- Imagine the recipient being engulfed in energy, see yourself doing a treatment on them, or simply empty your head and let the energy flow

Do some Experiments

In practice Distant Healing is sent for 10-15 minutes at a time, over a number of consecutive days, say 3-5 days. Have a friend sit down at a prearranged time each evening, in a quiet room, with their eyes closed and no distractions. Send Reiki at the time agreed and see what they noticed.

Distant Healing Books and Boxes

You can send Reiki to more than one person at a time. Have a book containing a list of people that you would like to send Reiki to. Review the list, draw HSZSN over the book, hold the book between your palms and Reiki the book with the intention that energy is being sent to all the recipients.

Use a box containing photographs - and names on pieces of paper - as an alternative. Draw HSZSN over the box and Reiki it with your hands.

Week 8 – Column 2

Send Reiki to the Past

Using HSZSN it is possible to focus Reiki on past events that have had an effect on how you think and feel about things. You can heal the effects that a difficult part of your life has had on you. Imagine the situation, visualise HSZSN over it, and send Reiki.

Send Reiki to the Future

It is possible to send Reiki out in advance, and it hangs around ready to deposit itself at the intended time, whether that be a particular time, or conditional on something happening. Send Reiki in advance to interviews or public speaking engagements. Send Reiki to your bed so that you receive it when you get into bed at night.

When you 'experiment' on someone, some days send Reiki in real time, on other days send it out in advance. See what happens.

Creative use of HSZSN

People send Reiki to world crises and conflicts like the Gulf War, the Kosovo crisis, to the victims and rescue workers at the World Trade Centre, or for general planetary healing.

Send Reiki to heal the relationship between two people, always with the proviso that it is for the highest good of the people involved. You are not imposing your preferred solution on the situation.

Ethics of Distant Healing

Some people think it is wrong to send Reiki to someone who hasn't asked for it. I disagree. Reiki is a beautiful healing energy that does not harm, you are sending the energy to the person's highest good, so you are not manipulating or imposing. Send Reiki to be received whenever is appropriate for the person.

Homework

Please carry on with your daily Hatsurei.

Find some willing victims to practice distant healing on, play around with the energy, and see what happens!

Week 9

The week 6 hand-out is not interesting in terms of layout.

Week 9 – Column 1

The Reiki Kotodama

This is just a little interesting information about Usui's method. When he taught people he gave them different ways that they could use to connect to the three energies. If his students were Buddhists then he gave them meditations; if they followed Shintoism then he gave them 'kotodama'. The word 'kotodama' means 'word spirit' or 'the soul of language' and these ancient Shinto mantras are said to represent different aspects of creation. They turn up in mystical Buddhism and martial arts, and there are historical accounts of these sounds being used to stop armies, to heal, to kill, and to control the weather. There is barely a handful of kotodama Masters in the whole of Japan now, and they reflect a tradition that disappears into the mists of ancient Japanese history.

Within Reiki, the kotodama were used to contact the energies that the symbols represent. They predate the use of symbols in Reiki, and it seems that they symbols were only introduced into Reiki in the last year of Usui's life, for the benefit of his students who could not get on with the other two approaches: Dr Hayashi and two other naval officers. Dr Hayashi taught Mrs Takata, and she passed on the 'symbol' tradition in the West.

Eye and Breath Techniques

In the original form of Reiki you were taught to send Reiki using your eyes and your breath. To send Reiki with your eyes, look with a loving state of being, use soft focus (defocus your eyes), stare through the place where you want to send Reiki, and intend that the energy passes with your gaze.

To send Reiki with your breath, put your tongue to the roof of your mouth, draw energy into your crown as you breathe in, and as you breathe out, still keeping your tongue in place, imagine that the energy passes with your breath.

These two techniques serve to demonstrate the power and importance of intent: you are not sending Reiki out of your eyes like Superman, but your visualisation focuses your intent in a particular way, and the energy takes on some of the connotations of staring and breathing. Reiki sent with the eyes seems more piercing, focused and precise, whereas Reiki sent with the breath seems more diffuse and superficial.

Week 9 – Column 2

Boosting the Flow of Energy

There is always some limit to how much energy can come through you, letting the energy flow of its own accord. No-one is a perfect channel. When you get to a 'hotspot', you can make the treatment more effective by boosting the flow of energy. You wouldn't want to use these methods all the way through a treatment, but just when you find a part of the body that's drawing lots of Reiki. Here are two techniques...

'Many Hands' technique

Imagine that you have a couple of extra sets of arms on each side, with additional hands either resting on top of your real ones, or in different treatment positions. Imagine energy flowing through the imaginary hands as well as the real ones. This will boost the flow of Reiki, and direct energy into the recipient's body from where the imaginary hands are.

The 'Hui Yin' circuit

There are a couple of special meridians that run down the midline of your body at the front and the back. They are called the Functional and Governor channels. If you connect up these meridians then Reiki is circulated around your body and is just vented through your hands

362

rather than leaking out elsewhere. This helps you to get the greatest benefit out of the energy that is coming into you.

Connect up this circuit when you get to a 'hotspot' and you will boost the flow of energy.

Connect the circuit by resting your tongue against the roof of your mouth, just behind the front teeth, and by pulling up your 'hui yin' point: your pelvic floor. Aim for a very gentle but definite contraction of a very small part of your anatomy, not an 'Arnold Schwarzenegger' contraction! Maintain this connection.

Homework

Please carry on with your daily Hatsurei, and make self-treatments a regular activity.

When you are treating someone, experiment with the 'energy boosting' techniques.

Week 10

The week 6 hand-out is not interesting in terms of layout.

Week 10 – Column 1

The Power of Intent

Intent underlies everything that we do with Reiki. We can make up complicated rituals, or do little visualisations, but all we are doing is focusing our intent in a particular way. Reiki is very simple: if you intend that the energy is sent in a particular way, or received in a particular way, then it is.

Beaming

You can 'fire' Reiki from one side of the room to another by sending it out of your palms, or your fingertips. Find a friend with a headache, sit them at the other end of the room, and beam Reiki through your hands to them. Beam your garden if you like!

Radiating

You can send Reiki out of your whole body, just radiate it. If someone is talking to you about one of their problems, feel yourself connecting to their thoughts and emotions and radiate Reiki out of your whole body to them. It is that simple. They will not be able to maintain their focus on the sad situation, it will seem more remote. They may even forget what it was that was making them feel down. You can try this with a friend as an experiment: just get them focus on a sad time in their life, and send Reiki to them.

A Final Word from Mikao Usui

…taken from the manual given to students of 'his' Society (Usui Reiki Ryoho Gakkai) in Japan…

Question:
Can anybody learn Usui Reiki Ryoho?

Answer:

"Of course, a man, woman, young or old, people with knowledge or without knowledge, anybody who has a common sense can receive the power accurately in a short time and can heal selves and others. I have taught to more than one thousand people but no one is failed. Everyone is able to heal illness with just Shoden (first degree). You may think it is inscrutable to get the healing power in a short time but it is reasonable. It is the feature of my method that heals difficult illnesses easily."

Week 10 – Column 2

Moving energy with intent

The energy follows your thought, it follows your focus. It will move where you want it to.

Imagine that you are doing a Western-style self-treatment. You have a back-ache. You can rest your hands on your front and imagine that Reiki is passing from your hands, through your body, to the area of need. It will do that.

Alternatively, draw the energy down through your crown and imagine it passing through your body to the areas of need. It will do that too.

If when you are treating someone you imagine that the energy is moving through their body to a particular part of their body, then it will do that.

If you are thinking nice warm thoughts about another person then *zoom*, Reiki will be following your thoughts and you will be sending distant Reiki without constructing any ritual.

It can be that simple!

So, What Happens Now?

Well, that is up to you. The more you work with Reiki, the greater the benefits that you will experience. Reiki will continue to make long-lasting positive changes in your life, it will occasionally give you a rough ride, and if you decide to work on others then you will be truly amazed by what it can do!

Beyond Second Degree level is Reiki Mastership. To move on to this level, you need to be comfortable with everything we have covered at 2nd Degree and had a chance to put it all into practice, and you need to feel ready to move on. Don't rush the process. Enjoy the journey.

Homework

You are now well equipped to work with Reiki!

Get lots of practice until you are comfortable with the techniques that we have talked about, and find your own way of working with the energy.

Good luck, and keep in touch!

Sample Evening Class Session

To help you get to grips with organising your own session, here is how I put my sessions together.

The evening classes lasted for 2 hours each time, with a break for about 10 minutes or so half way through. After the first session, each week we began by getting feedback from the students:

- How had their homework gone?
- How do they feel within themselves?
- What feedback did they get from anyone the practised on?

Then I would talk about one aspect of Reiki for a while, and then move on to give everyone Reiju empowerments.

We would take some feedback from people to see what they noticed, and then we would break for 10 minutes.

For the second session we would start with my introducing some practical exercises for them to do, on their own or in pairs or small groups.

Students would give their feedback as we went along or at the end of the session, and the evening would finish with me telling them what their homework would be, and giving them their weekly handout.

So, for example, weeks #2 and #3 of the course went like this:

Evening Classes: Session # 2

Part One

10 mins	Homework Feedback
20 mins	Talk: The effects of Attunements and Self-treatment
20 mins	Give Reiju empowerments Feedback
<BREAK>	10 mins

Part Two

25 mins	Self-Treatment meditation
25 mins	Hatsurei Ho
Homework	Hatsurei The Self-Treatment Meditation

Evening Classes: Session # 3

Part One

10 mins   Homework Feedback

20 mins   Talk:
                 What it's like to give and
                 Receive Reiki

20 mins   Give Reiju empowerments
                 Feedback

\<BREAK\>   10 mins

Part Two

In pairs:

25 mins   Feel the energy field, scan, and
                 Give a seated Reiki treatment

Swap over, and...

25 mins   Feel the energy field, scan, and
                 Give a seated Reiki treatment

Homework   Hatsurei
                 The Self-Treatment Meditation

Lightning Source UK Ltd.
Milton Keynes UK
UKOW04f1807301017
311907UK00001B/85/P